to tend & to hold

to tend & to hold

Honoring Our Bodies, Our Needs, and Our Grief Through Pregnancy and Infant Loss

Eileen S. Rosete

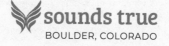

sounds true
BOULDER, COLORADO

Sounds True
Boulder, CO

This book is not intended as a substitute for the medical recommendations of physicians, mental health professionals, or other health-care providers. Rather, it is intended to offer information to help the reader cooperate with physicians, mental health professionals, and health-care providers in a mutual quest for optimal well-being. We advise readers to carefully review and understand the ideas presented and to seek the advice of a qualified professional before attempting to use them.

Published 2024

Book design by Charli Barnes
Illustrations © 2024 Jo Situ Allen

Printed in Canada

BK06369

Library of Congress Cataloging-in-Publication Data

Names: Rosete, Eileen S., author.
Title: To tend and to hold : honoring our bodies, our needs, and our grief through pregnancy
    and infant loss / Eileen S. Rosete.
Description: Boulder, CO : Sounds True, Inc., 2024. | Includes bibliographical references.
Identifiers: LCCN 2024007597 (print) | LCCN 2024007598 (ebook) | ISBN
    9781683648956 (hardback) | ISBN 9781683648963 (ebook)
Subjects: LCSH: Miscarriage--Psychological aspects. | Newborn infants--
    Death--Psychological aspects. | Stillbirth--Psychological aspects. | Grief.
    | Postnatal care.
Classification: LCC RG648 .R64 2024 (print) | LCC RG648 (ebook) |
    DDC 618.3/92--dc23/eng/20240520
LC record available at https://lccn.loc.gov/2024007597
LC ebook record available at https://lccn.loc.gov/2024007598

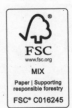

FSC
www.fsc.org
MIX
Paper | Supporting
responsible forestry
FSC® C016245

For all who know the depths of pregnancy and infant loss.

May you feel seen. May you feel heard. May you feel held.

Here and across the veil.

May you be known.

To Tend and To Hold

To Tend and To Hold is an offering made in love especially for you, dear reader. You who have, are currently, or will soon be enduring pregnancy loss or infant loss—what I often refer to as *womb loss*. It is an offering made with the deepest reverence for the demands that those of us who conceive, gestate, and birth come to know deep in our being whether we birth life, death, or both.

To tend is to offer attention and care to something or someone with gentleness and loving intention. The idea of tending became prominent in the course of writing this book as I centered those of us who have experienced the ending of a pregnancy or the death of a fetus in our bodies or soon after giving birth. So much of what it means to grieve and heal from a loss as embodied as ours is bringing loving attention and intention to the parts of us that are hurting. I also came to apply these words in a self-generative way as the pandemic revealed the importance of being able to resource oneself when external sources of support may be difficult to access. I call this *self-tending*. More than the phrase self-care, self-tending feels softer, gentler, and doable. Self-tending is about caring for yourself at your own pace and in your own way. It is also about honoring your current capacity by doing only as much as you are able to in any given moment and knowing that is enough. At its essence, self-tending is simply being gentle with yourself.

To hold is to take into one's hands or arms, to support, and to contain. To feel held is to feel comforted and safe to soften. This book is here to hold you. So that you can feel comforted. So that you can feel safe to soften your guard and your body. For it is in such softening that we can hear our deepest needs and then be able to tend to them.

I write these words to you in the midst of my favorite part of the day: the late afternoon, just before the California sun descends fully into the horizon. I love seeing how the sun's golden glow embraces the space around me. And I love feeling its gentle rays on my skin. In moments such as this, I often close my eyes and receive the tending the sun has to offer, allowing its warmth to sink in and ease the tension I carry. In such moments, I feel held—warmed, comforted, safe. And this is what I hope for you. That you may feel both tended to and held, knowing that such felt experiences can be of your own making as well as a response to care from others or the healing power of Mother Nature. This book exists through the efforts of countless individuals who want this for you, too, and who are working devotedly to create a world that cares for and honors all who experience womb loss. Know that we deserve a world that recognizes our loss as real, our grief as valid, and our postpartum healing as worthy of support.[1] May you feel the truth in this and may the world know it.

Womb and Womb Loss

Known also as the uterus, the womb is an incredibly unique and highly dynamic muscular organ that is vital to menstruation, fertility, pregnancy, labor, and birth.[1] In the menstrual cycle, the womb continuously builds and sheds a thick, spongy lining of blood and tissue, meant to be a soft, nurturing place for a fertilized egg to land and grow.[2] In pregnancy, the womb, which was previously hollow, endures profound structural and cellular shifts to carry all that will call it home: blastocysts, embryos, and later fetuses (living and nonliving), empty gestational sacs (if embryos do not develop), and the placenta—an entirely new organ that the body grows to provide nutrients and oxygen to a fetus while removing waste and carbon dioxide through the umbilical cord.[3] Remarkably, the uterus can stretch from the size of a lemon to that of a watermelon to hold a growing fetus, a growing placenta, a growing umbilical cord, and increased amniotic fluid.[4] In labor, the uterine muscles contract powerfully to encourage all that is held within to leave the body through the vagina. After birth, whether vaginally or through a procedure, there is a significant internal wound where the placenta was previously attached to the uterine wall, yet the womb continues to exert itself by contracting for an estimated six weeks to release lochia (blood, mucus, and uterine tissue) and return to a nonpregnant state in a process called uterine involution.[5] It takes extraordinary endurance and resilience to do what the womb does. To do what you do. And it is time to afford both the respect and reverence they deserve.

The phrase *womb loss* is used in this book to describe all forms of pregnancy loss at any point of gestation and infant loss. I first came across it in the work of women's health physical therapist and acclaimed author Tami Lynn Kent. I share it here as a way to center those of us who have endured pregnancy and infant loss by locating such loss explicitly within and of our bodies. Because you deserve to be centered. You deserve to be known.

Contents

A Moment of Silence

Before we begin, I invite you to pause for a moment of silence to honor yourself and your experience of womb loss. For they are deserving of such a moment.

If it feels resonant, place one or both hands over your heart and either soften your gaze or close your eyes. Allow the silence to last as long as you need it to. Maybe for just a few breaths, maybe for a few minutes.

And as you take this moment to be in silence, you might consider all those who are also holding this book and doing so alongside you. You are not alone in your pain.

When you are ready, allow your breath to help return you to the present, slowly opening your eyes if they are closed.

And it is with this spirit of reverence that we begin.

Introduction

Your Loss Is Our Loss

I am so sorry for your loss, and all you've had to endure.
And all you continue to endure.

As I write this, I am feeling into my own losses, and even years later, the feelings that overwhelmed me then are with me now, just beneath the surface. Less intense, yet ever present. The body remembers those experiences that leave such deep impressions.

Whether your pregnancy was wanted, unwanted, or somewhere in between. Whether the pregnancy ended in the first trimester, second, or third, or if your infant was born alive and died soon after. Whether you have children who are living or only across the veil. And whether your loss was recent, in the last few years, decades ago, or has yet to transpire. However you came to hold this book in your hands, I am sorry for the pain that brought you here, and I offer you my heartfelt sympathy. For your loss is real. Your grief is valid. And you deserve the deepest of condolences. No matter how much time has passed between my writing these words and your reading of them, know that my heart aches with you.

A Story of Comfort

In the summer of 2017, just a few weeks after experiencing my second pregnancy loss, I found myself walking down the hall of a small, single-story office suite in Redlands, California. I felt a little anxious as I followed the massage therapist, despite her coming highly recommended by my chiropractor. The space was unfamiliar, the massage therapist was new to me, and I was feeling tender physically and emotionally.

In our text exchange before my appointment, I felt an intuitive pull to share that I had just experienced a pregnancy loss. In addition to being a massage therapist, Heather was a birth doula and in training to become a midwife. I wanted her to know that I was in a fragile state and figured she, of all people, would understand how to care for someone like me—someone who was both postpartum and bereaved.

The moment I crossed the threshold into her space, my body felt at ease, and I knew I was where I needed to be. The small room was bathed in a welcoming darkness save for the peaceful glow of candlelight and a salt lamp. The sounds of soft instrumental music added to the sense of calm, and the walls were decorated with artwork celebrating pregnancy and motherhood. While seeing this could have easily been a painful reminder of my no longer being pregnant, I instead felt reassured that I was with someone who would understand my postbirth body.

Left alone to undress, I sighed as I settled in between the soft sheets warmed by the heated massage table. Then, after gently knocking on the door and hearing I was ready, Heather approached with a tiny bottle in hand. Uncapping it, she brought the bottle closer and asked if I'd like her to use this essential oil she had picked out with my pregnancy loss in mind. I was surprised by the thoughtful gesture and said yes to the floral scent.

She added a few drops to the carrier oil in her palm, and as soon as her hands pressed onto my skin and I inhaled the sweet aroma of ylang-ylang, my eyes filled with tears and my body softened to her firm yet reverent touch. The intention infused into the essential oil and Heather's deferential mien deepened the experience from a massage to a moment of witnessing. And though I lay quiet, my tired body told her its story, relieved to have someone who could understand, each knot of tense muscle testifying to all that I still carried despite my womb being empty.

As Heather's hands glided, kneaded, and pressed deeply into each of these knots, I breathed into the discomfort and the pain until together we helped my body release what it had been holding. It was as if my body had stored some of my most difficult emotions and memories until I had the capacity and support to face them. As if my body, wise in and of itself, knew I couldn't face the entirety of my grief all at once nor on my own. I found the relief I had been longing for, and with that relief, my postbirth body was finally able to rest.

~

It has been many years since that initial session with Heather. Still, whenever I smell ylang-ylang, I return to that morning. My mind remembers the details of a room that felt like a sanctuary. My body remembers how it felt to be tended to with such care. At a time when it was so hard for me to be in my body, the site of my trauma, Heather helped me know relief was possible.

This is what I wish for you, dear reader, that you too may know what it feels like to be seen, heard, and held with respect and reverence. And that you may feel moments of relief even amidst your pain. You are deserving of such felt experiences. And they are essential to grieving and postpartum healing alike.

Not one person or thing can fully ease or take away the thoughts, feelings, and sensations you are experiencing. Such healing is yours to tend to, in your own time and in your own way. But you don't have to do it alone. Nor should you have to. You have been through so much already.

So, whether you offer yourself a massage or other acts of care, know you are worthy of feeling comforted and worthy of feeling relief. So that you may rest. So that you may have the fortitude to face each moment as it comes.

It Began with a Vision

A year after my session with Heather, a vision came to me, one that was as detailed as it was powerful. In it, I saw a group of women gathered around a small body of water, the night simplifying their surroundings with a blanket of darkness. Some stood with their arms wrapped around themselves. Others stood arm in arm with a neighbor, gently leaning into one another for warmth and support.

Their solemn expressions were illuminated partly by moonlight, partly by starlight, and partly by the soft glow of numerous candles floating on the water before them. As the candles gently swayed, the women stood still, looking at and through the flames into memories—some recent, some more distant. The silence was heavy with all that was felt but unsaid.

I carried an intuitive knowing that these women had gathered to honor their pregnancy losses and the babies they could not hold. Just as importantly, they had come to honor themselves, what they had experienced, and the fact that they had survived.

There was a candle for each of them and a candle for each of their womb losses, flames testifying to deep wounds otherwise unseen, to hard-earned resilience unacknowledged until then, and to an invisible community of grievers.

~

After receiving this vision, I began to long deeply for such a gathering for myself and others who had survived pregnancy and infant loss. To acknowledge our shared pain, to mourn openly and honestly without inhibition, and to honor what we and our bodies had gone through. All without feeling the need to explain or justify ourselves. The universe seemed to agree as things fell into place with extraordinary ease, and I hosted my first event that fall.

The first Our Womb Loss dining event was an elevated, intimate gathering I will always remember. Held in a stunning home tucked away from the busy streets of West Los Angeles, my guests and I sat around a dining table beautifully set with earth-toned linen, stoneware plates, tea lights, and flowers. Menus resting on our napkins gave us a preview of the delicious postpartum food being carefully prepared by the head chef of MotherBees (a Los Angeles-based postpartum food delivery service turned global motherhood support platform) just a few feet away. I gazed at my guests through teary eyes and shared why this event came to be—that our womb losses were important enough to recognize and that we who carried such loss with our bodies deserved to be honored with intention, beauty, and love. Each person shared their name and what brought them to the table that evening. We listened to stories of loss as well as current struggles. And we heard many repeat the desire to finally make time for themselves. We listened, and we witnessed, holding space by giving our full attention to every speaker without interruption. Later, as the chef introduced each finely plated dish, Heng Ou, founder of MotherBees and author of the seminal postpartum book *The First Forty Days: The Art of Nourishing the New Mother*, explained in detail how each was deeply nourishing for the postpartum body, including our bodies that were postpartum after womb loss.

After dinner and under the light of a full moon, we walked in shared silence to the pool in the backyard, where we placed floating LED candles into the water—one for ourselves and one for each of our losses. As the last candle was set into the water, the scene in front of me merged with the one I had seen in my mind and carried close to my heart: a group of women standing around a small body of water. Some stood with their arms wrapped around themselves. Others stood arm in arm with a neighbor, gently leaning into one another for warmth and support. Their solemn expressions illuminated partly by moonlight, partly by the pool's lights, and partly by the soft glow of numerous candles floating on the water before them. As the candles gently swayed, the women stood still, looking at and through the flames into memories—some recent, some more distant. The silence was heavy with all that was felt but unsaid.

By the time I hosted my third Our Womb Loss event a year later, I knew I wanted to capture the essence of these gatherings in a book that could help others feel the way my guests felt: seen, heard, held, and honored. I said as much at the dinner table that memorable evening in October 2019, knowing that speaking it aloud could help bring it into being. And it did.

A Soft Place to Land

To Tend and To Hold is a refuge for all who have experienced loss during or after their pregnancy, as well as those who are currently pregnant and anticipating loss or are living through it in this very moment. For all who feel grief for the womb loss they've endured, may this book be a soft place for you to land.

This may include those who experienced loss before or during birth or those who experienced loss after birthing a living child. This may include those whose bodies released the pregnancy on their own or those whose bodies needed medication or a proceedure to do so. This may include those whose pregnancies did not lead to a growing embryo or fetus or those whose bodies could conceive and carry a pregnancy only with the support of fertility treatment. This may include those who also have living children or those whose only children are beyond touch. This may include those whose pregnancies ended with the birth of living, thriving children *and* loss, such as in adoption (the baby going to a foster or adoptive family), surrogacy (the baby being united with their intended parents), or pregnancy with multiples (as with vanishing twin syndrome). This may include those who have experienced womb loss once or those who have known it many times over.

There are so many manifestations of pregnancy and infant loss, and truly no right or wrong way to feel about your lived experience of it. Whatever you are feeling is valid. What matters most is what your womb loss means to you. Maybe you carry multiple, seemingly contradictory feelings about your experience. Maybe you're not sure how or what to feel. For some, the experience may be more about the physicality of healing their postpartum bodies, while others may feel the need to process the physical, mental, emotional, spiritual, or relational impact of their womb loss. For some, it is but one part of their lives; for others it is life-altering.

However womb loss looks and feels for you, this book is meant to meet you where you are. To welcome and hold space for you. With kindness. Without judgment or expectation.

There is room for all of us to be named and to be known.

How to Use This Book

I bring myself to these pages in the midst of my fifth postpartum season. Writing this book as I am acutely postpartum has been difficult. It is hard to do much of anything after conceiving, gestating, and birthing. No matter the length of gestation, all these processes take a toll on the body, and for many of us, on the heart. And yet, such timing has allowed me to write about postpartum needs from a deeply embodied place. It has also allowed me to better access the depths of the grief and trauma I still carry from my womb losses, despite the years and the living children who have come since then. The result is a book that holds space for the tender intersection of postpartum care, grief, and trauma. One that meets you where you are with the deepest compassion—whether years, months, weeks, or days from your loss, or whether you are still pregnant—and honors that we are all postpartum when our pregnancies come to an end at any point in gestation.

To Tend and To Hold is divided into three parts: "Our Loss," "Our Grief," and "Our Healing." Part 1, "Our Loss," invites you to consider three significant, though often overlooked, thresholds: when you learn about your womb loss, when you birth your loss, and the time immediately after when you begin to endure your loss as both postpartum and bereaved. Part 2, "Our Grief," is dedicated to addressing grief in the context of womb loss, including the intersection of grief and trauma, our loved ones and their grief, and mourning our loss and ourselves. Part 3, "Our Healing," delves deeper into long-term postpartum care after womb loss, how to support survivors of such loss (yourself and others), and what you might consider for life ahead.

Each chapter contains a carefully curated collection of stories, essential information, nourishing postpartum recipes, and gentle embodiment practices. The stories shared are meant to offer comfort and show you what is possible for your healing process. You will not find traumatic stories of pregnancy and infant loss detailed here, for in my grief, I found it too hard to read such accounts. My trauma felt like enough to carry. However, if you feel drawn to read other stories of womb loss, you will find a list of thoughtfully chosen memoirs in the resources section.

The information shared here is meant to help you make informed decisions when it is so easy to feel adrift, alone, and unsure. This is information I and many other womb loss survivors wish we had. We want so much for you to know your options, to choose what best serves you and your needs, and to live lives that are meaningful to you—lives that integrate your grief rather than lives constrained by it.

Each chapter shares a postpartum recipe I personally love and prepare for myself, friends, and my postpartum doula clients. It can be hard to tend to our basic needs when we are exhausted from pregnancy and birth, overwhelmed with grief, and burdened with trauma, so I have chosen simple recipes with few ingredients and easy-to-follow steps. They are also nutrient-rich to aid in your body's transition from pregnancy. Even if it has been many months or years since you birthed your loss, know that your body is forever postpartum and can benefit from food and drink that support it and your well-being.

Each chapter offers several embodiment practices. They are gentle invitations to connect intentionally with your breath, mind, body, spirit, and relationships. If it ever becomes difficult to be with thoughts, feelings, or physical sensations that arise, these simple practices can help you feel grounded and more able to endure moments of struggle. They are practices you can take with you and turn to long after you've closed this book.

You will also find a special section entitled "Offering from the Collective" toward the end of each chapter. These are loving contributions from health professionals and healing arts practitioners, many of whom are beloved friends who have supported me through my fertility journey. Each offering briefly describes a particular healing modality, how it can support survivors of womb loss, and a simple self-tending practice that you can add to your repertoire. These practices were created specifically with you in mind, dear reader, so that you may feel seen, held, and honored. For you are deserving of all these things. Know that you can turn to these self-tending practices whenever your body longs for well-deserved tenderness.

Finally, each chapter concludes with a short reflection on the content we covered and a closing verse that is repeated throughout the book. This verse is an invitation to acknowledge where and how you are in that moment with compassion and to feel held by the collective response that follows.

~

In the spirit of being trauma sensitive, as womb loss can feel incredibly traumatic for many, this book acknowledges that you are the expert of your body, and as such, you know best what is needed for your healing—though coming to such a place of self-awareness may take time, effort, and the support of others. Know that everything here is an invitation. The following are a few such invitations to support you as you read on:

Go to what calls you. This book does not need to be read in any particular order. Allow yourself to go to what feels most resonant in a given moment.

Honor your own pace. If at any point you feel overwhelmed or notice your body responding in a way that feels uncomfortable or even painful, consider taking a moment to pause and do something that feels grounding before moving on or put the book down and take a break.

Choose what feels right. We can so often feel helpless amidst womb loss, when our ability to choose is taken away, when what choices we do have don't feel like choices at all, or when it's not clear what our options are and no one is there to guide us. This book is designed to honor your agency by using invitational language and offering options.

Notice what feels resonant. This may feel like an internal "YES!"—a sensation of being pulled toward the page or a desire to underline or highlight what you just read. It can be tearing up or crying. It can feel like a softening of the shoulders, a sense of affirmation when something on the page speaks to a deep truth within you. You might give yourself a moment to stay in that response and allow what is emerging to express itself more fully.

Make it yours. While ancestral wisdom and modern guidelines for grieving and postpartum care do exist, both are processes with no definitive course or clear end. Let your process of grieving and your process of postpartum healing be just that: *yours.* Draw inspiration from what already exists and also allow yourself to follow your intuition.

Honor your innate resilience. At the heart of *To Tend and To Hold* is a foundational belief in your innate resilience—your capacity to endure and adapt after experiencing hardship. In moments of struggle, simply allowing yourself to take your next breath is a powerful act of resilience. It truly is. So know this and call on the resilient part of you when you are in need.

If You Are in Crisis

It is natural to long for relief from the pain of womb loss, to be utterly desperate for it. How can we be in this world if each day, each moment, feels unbearable? And yet, relief can come. And it can manifest in many different forms.

Sadly, death by suicide is the leading cause of maternal mortality during pregnancy until one year after birth (also referred to as *perinatal suicide*), with most deaths occurring in the postpartum period. Globally, perinatal suicide accounts for up to 20 percent of postpartum deaths, and in the US, rates of suicidal ideation during pregnancy increased by 100 percent from 2008 to 2018, with Black birthing people experiencing the largest increase in rates by 700 percent.[1] Despite such dire statistics, research on the topic is nascent, and there is an urgent, unmet need for evidence-based strategies to prevent it.[2]

If you have intentions or actionable plans for self-harm or suicide or have already made attempts, please know there is support for you. Self-harm or death by suicide is not the only way to find the relief you seek. I encourage you to put this book down for now and call your local emergency number, a national crisis and suicide hotline, or someone in your life you can trust to be of help—be it a therapist or other health-care professional, a partner, a friend, or a family member. Consider creating a safety plan to clarify what would feel truly helpful to you, and keep it on the fridge or another place that is easily accessible. You don't need to endure these moments of struggle alone. Nor should you have to. You have been through so much already.

~

The following three embodiment practices were shared with me when I was writing from the desert lands of southern Utah en route to a run/walk for pregnancy and infant loss in Calgary, Alberta, Canada. As it happens with souls you feel like you were meant to meet, Teána and I felt an instant connection, and our conversation deepened into talk of her struggles, including with fertility and suicide. It was clear she had worked hard to gain the peace and clarity with which she spoke of such hard things. She also listened with a generous heart as I read aloud the passage above, and shared practices she wished someone had given her for her greatest times of need. I offer them here with her beautiful, resilient spirit in mind and hope they can be of service to you.

- Go outside and find a leaf. Crumple it in your hands and notice the sensations.

- Stand outside and just focus on the feeling of the sun warming your body.

- Tap your body with your fingertips, especially the parts of you that feel numb.

Living with the pain of womb loss is possible. There are many who can attest to this, and we hope you stay with us.

Your Healing Is Our Healing

Your loss is our loss. Though we have experienced different types of womb loss. Though our timelines may differ—some of us closer or further from the period of acute grief. Though we may be in different parts of the world, from different backgrounds, and of different identities. A loss as intimate as womb loss has the power to transcend it all and connect us through our common humanity.

And your healing is our healing. We who have lived and continue to live into our unique processes of grieving and postpartum healing are here to hold you and hold space for you. We who have survived and are able to thrive once more hope that you will too, in your own time and in your own way. Notice the "our" in *your*, and know we are in this together. You are not alone. We are with you.

Terminology

A Softer Shared Language

You deserve softness.

Late one night, years after experiencing my womb losses, I came across an online essay by Motherly that shifted something deep inside me. In this powerfully heartfelt and heartbreaking letter from a mother to her unborn child, the author writes:

> The English language refers to the incident as a "miscarriage." The Filipino and Bicol languages, on the other hand, labeled me as a woman with an unborn child, as "nakunan/nakuanan." These roughly translate into "someone from whom something was taken away."[1]

The moment I read this, it was as if time stopped. Despite being the daughter of Filipino immigrants, immersed in the sounds of my family's mix of English and Tagalog, these terms were new to me. And yet these words spoke to a deep truth within me.

My doctors and midwives reassured me that, as with the majority of early pregnancy losses, my losses were likely due to chromosomal abnormalities and therefore beyond my control. Yet part of me still carried feelings of remorse since it was my body that had been carrying these pregnancies, and because it was my body, it seemed there was more I could have done.

The language used to describe my kind of loss seemed to imply as much and that the onus lay solely with me, especially with the prefix *mis-* (meaning "wrongly or badly"):

| Miscarriage | Miscarried | Lost |
| *I had a miscarriage.* | *I miscarried.* | *I lost my babies.* |

As if I had made a *mis*take when I had a *mis*carriage. As if I had done something bad when I *mis*carried. As if I had been irresponsible or absent-minded when I *lost* my babies. As if they could be found if I just tried hard enough, though they were in my body all along.

When I found this essay—or when it found me—I sat staring at it for a long moment, and in that pause, the part of me that carried remorse came to the surface. She read and re-read those three sentences, awed that such words existed to describe her. Awed by what felt like a gentle reframing of her loss.

She, too, was *nakunan*. I, too, was *nakuanan*.

In these words we felt seen. We felt known. And with that we felt relief as the edges of our remorse softened. I was and am someone with unborn children. I was and am someone from whom something was taken away. These words from the languages of my ancestors found me and held me when my native tongue seemed to blame me. It was a powerful, quiet moment that left a deep impression.

~

What I felt then, I hope you, dear reader, can feel too. For all who have experienced womb loss in their bodies, with their bodies, deserve a softer shared language that evokes compassion rather than shame. That validates rather than stigmatizes. That invites healing connection rather than isolation.

Your womb loss was something you experienced. It is something that happened to you and your body. You are someone from whom something was taken away.

There is no international consensus on language to describe womb loss during and after pregnancy. It may surprise you to learn that this, which seems so basic, is missing. As it stands, terminology varies across and even within countries. Terms used in the press and in policy differ from those used in medical writing. That a standardized vocabulary does not exist makes it difficult to communicate clearly. Between health-care providers and patients. Among health-care providers themselves. Between the media and the public. Among those who have decision-making powers and whose decisions shape the contexts in which we experience womb loss. The lack of a shared language also hampers research efforts, making it difficult to collect and compare data. It also makes it hard for those of us trying to name and understand our lived experience of womb loss, leaving many feeling confused, unsure, blamed, and ashamed. And the terms that *are* commonly used can often feel at odds with the felt experience and descriptors used by those of us who survive womb loss.

But language is ever evolving, and we do not need to settle for what is (and what is not). While the lack of a standardized lexicon for womb loss speaks to the subjectivity of terms, it also points to the potential for something new. As the Motherly essay shows us, there are other ways to talk about womb loss, and we can in fact define our experiences for ourselves by choosing to use words that feel respectful and true to us, or by creating the language we're longing for. Language that engenders dignity. Language that conveys empathy. A vocabulary that invites our shared humanity into the conversation.

This book seeks to embody such a language and to encourage language that is more clear and literal. While it is common to see, hear, and use euphemisms like "passed away," "the baby is sleeping," or "we lost the baby," especially in cultures that are death-averse and shy away from words like *death* and *died,* this can cause confusion. Such distinctions are especially important when talking to living children who are enduring this loss along-side you. They may wonder when the baby will wake up or feel afraid that anyone who falls asleep (themselves included) may not wake up again. They may also wonder where the baby is and what can be done to find them. The baby who has died cannot wake up, and while you have experienced a pro-found *loss*, you have not *lost* something that can be found.

Naming your experience can feel like a powerful affirmation, especially if your experience does not fall easily into commonly-known categories. In addition to those often used, below you will find terms that invite a softer, kinder conversation about womb loss in its different manifestations.

Terms That Can Be Used to Describe Pregnancy and Infant Loss by Gestational Age (GA)

<14 Weeks GA	≥14 Weeks GA	≥20 Weeks GA to Birth	After Birth
Anembryonic pregnancy[2] Biochemical pregnancy[2] Ectopic pregnancy Molar pregnancy[3] Embryonic death/ embryo loss First trimester pregnancy loss Early pregnancy loss/ early miscarriage	Second trimester pregnancy loss (14–27 weeks and 6 days GA) Second trimester miscarriage	Stillbirth/ intrauterine fetal demise (IUFD) Early stillbirth (20–27 weeks GA) Late stillbirth (28–36 weeks GA) Term stillbirth (≥37 weeks GA) Third trimester pregnancy loss (≥28 weeks GA)	Neonatal death (<28 days old) Infant death (<1 year old) Sudden infant death syndrome (SIDS <1 year old)
Miscarriage/spontaneous abortion Asymptomatic pregnancy loss/missed miscarriage/missed abortion Incomplete pregnancy loss/incomplete miscarriage/incomplete abortion Multifetal pregnancy reduction			
Fetal death/fetal loss (≥11 weeks GA) Induced abortion/medication abortion/abortion procedure Therapeutic abortion/therapeutic termination of pregnancy (TToP)/termination for medical reasons (TFMR)			
Pregnancy loss Induced pregnancy loss Recurrent pregnancy Loss			Infant loss
Perinatal loss (between conception to 28 days after birth) Baby loss Womb loss			

Note that this chart is based on gestational age (GA), which is calculated as the time since the first day of the last menstrual period (LMP), whereas most research on human development uses fertilization age, which, as the name implies, is the time since fertilization. Gestational age begins dating a pregnancy two weeks before fertilization actually occurs. This leaves a two-week difference between gestational age and fertilization age.

Again, definitions vary, as is the case with the term *stillbirth*. As seen above, *stillbirth* in the United States is commonly used to refer to pregnancy loss at or after 20 weeks of gestation, though in clinical practice, *early stillbirth* (20 to 27 weeks GA), *late stillbirth* (28 to 36 weeks GA), and *term stillbirth* (≥37 weeks GA) are the terms commonly used.[4] In the United Kingdom, the National Health Service (NHS) defines *stillbirth* as "when a baby is born dead after 24 completed weeks of pregnancy."[5] The World Health Organization, on the other hand, applies the term *stillbirth* to "a baby who dies after 28 weeks of pregnancy, but before or during birth."[6] Because terms and their definitions differ, it is useful to know what is being used where you live and by your health-care providers so that you can better understand your experience of womb loss and your options for care. Ask questions to clarify the terms and their meanings.

~

For the purposes of this book, the terms *womb loss* and *pregnancy and infant loss* are used interchangeably and refer to all forms of loss during pregnancy or after birth. This way, we have terms that honor our myriad experiences and validate all of our losses. With that in mind, know that there are many ways you can describe your unique experience of womb loss. Choose and use language that feels right for you. You might want to use words and phrases that refer to your pregnancy and pregnancy loss, or you might want to use ones that refer to your baby and baby loss. You may feel drawn to use a mix of both. Below are some examples. Choose what feels right for you in this moment. Use language that may not be included here and know that your preferences may shift over time.

My pregnancy . . .	My baby . . .
My pregnancy ended early.	My baby/babies died.
My pregnancy ended in the first trimester.	My baby died in utero.
My pregnancy ended in the second trimester.	My baby died in the womb.
My pregnancy ended in the third trimester.	My baby died in my body.
My pregnancy ended in loss.	My baby died in the first trimester.
My pregnancy ended in miscarriage.	My baby died in the second trimester.
My pregnancy ended in stillbirth.	My baby died in the third trimester.
My pregnancy ended in infant loss.	My baby died during labor.
My pregnancy was interrupted.	My baby died after birth.
	My baby was born dead.
I experienced womb loss.	I experienced the death of my baby during/after pregnancy.
I experienced pregnancy loss.	I experienced the loss of my baby during/after pregnancy.
I experienced an induced pregnancy loss.	I experienced baby loss.
I experienced the loss of a nonviable pregnancy.	I experienced infant loss.
I experienced a miscarriage.	
I experienced a stillbirth.	

You might choose to use alternate descriptors that speak more clearly to the challenges of your felt experience. For example, you might say, "I suffered a pregnancy loss," rather than "I experienced a pregnancy loss" to more aptly communicate your pain. You might even add another descriptor to more authentically convey your felt experience. For example, instead of "I suffered a pregnancy loss," you might say, "I suffered a traumatic pregnancy loss." Or you might say, "I'm a pregnancy loss survivor" to bring attention to the fact that pregnancy and pregnancy loss can take a tremendous toll on the body and come with many risks, even death, for those birthing. Use your intuition as you explore how to name what you've endured and how you feel. You can choose what words speak most truthfully to your felt experience. With the invitation for a softer shared language in mind, are there any words or phrases you would add to those shared in this section?

Many experience womb loss as a traumatic event, and terms such as *birth trauma, reproductive trauma,* or *medical trauma* may feel aligned with their felt experience. Often when talking about trauma, the words *trigger* and *triggered* are used to describe when a person encounters a stimulus that is associated with their trauma history and experiences a strong emotional and physical reaction. In keeping with the intention for a softer shared language, you will see the words *activate* and *activated* used here instead.

Words are powerful, and the labeling of one's experiences can have profound meaning and consequences. This is especially so for those who live in places where certain forms of pregnancy loss are criminalized and where health care to manage pregnancy loss is more difficult to access. Even in such situations, know that you can decide how to define your womb loss. You can choose designations that resonate most truthfully with your unique experience. With a softer shared language, may our world be better equipped to talk about womb loss with the reverence it deserves and to support those of us who endure it.

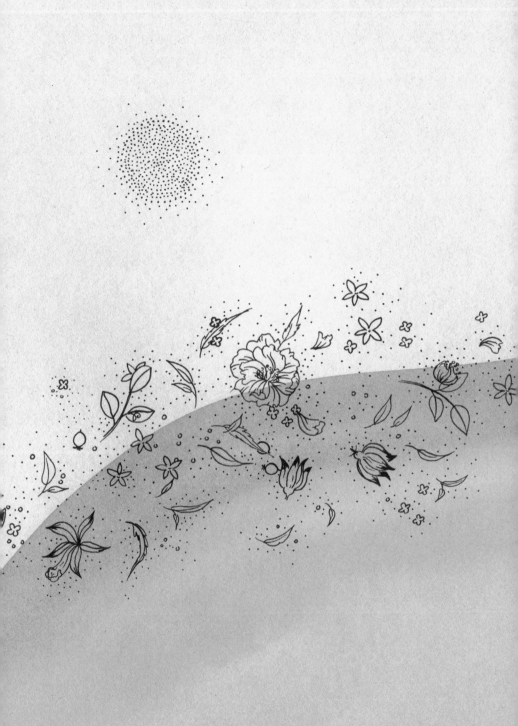

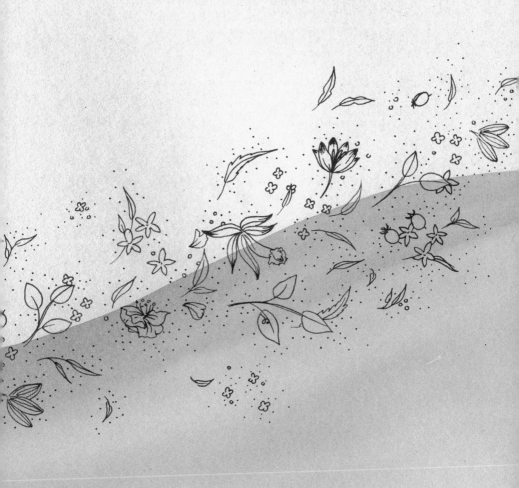

part one

our loss

CHAPTER 1

Learning About Your Loss

It's okay to cry.

I learned that I had experienced my first pregnancy loss during a routine ultrasound at what was supposed to be the first of many prenatal appointments. While the years and my grieving since have softened the pain of that morning, I clearly remember the moment my doctor's demeanor shifted during the ultrasound: from friendly and relaxed, to focused and concerned, to somber and apologetic. How she turned to me with sadness in her eyes and told me in the gentlest voice, "I'm so sorry, but there's no heartbeat." How her eyes held mine as I registered the news before folding over in tears. How she stood nearby holding space for me—silent, unrushed, and unwavering. She stepped out of the room at some point, letting me know she wanted to give me time alone and that she would be back in a few minutes. When she returned, she exuded only gentleness as she patiently explained options for supporting my body in releasing the pregnancy, and then she gave me time alone once again to consider them.

~

My doctor's warm bedside manner, gentle tone of voice, and willingness to companion me through the sudden and unexpected transition from expectant to bereaved mother left a lasting impression. Despite the agony I felt at the time and all the years that have passed, when I think back to that moment, what I feel most is comforted. It was a hard moment, *and* I was held through it. My body's response to this memory reminds me this was so.

Months and a move later, in the throes of my second pregnancy loss, I came to learn that not all who work with pregnancy are equipped to hold space for loss. It deepened my appreciation for the doctor who supported me the first time. She showed me what sensitive, respectful care can look like for those of us who birth loss and what all who experience womb loss deserve.

Learning that your pregnancy has ended in loss, may end in loss, or will inevitably end in loss is a tremendous moment, one that is layered and complex and deserves to be recognized for the immense threshold that it is. Thresholds are doorways, powerful moments of transition, with a distinct feeling of "before" and "after." Those of us who know womb loss understand the magnitude of this particular threshold, when we step into a completely different pregnancy experience than we expected, one that requires a whole new set of information and tools. No matter if your womb loss happened years ago, recently, or has yet to happen physically, I hope the information and practices here can support you as you process this moment of moments.

You Are Not Alone

For as long as there has been life, there has been death. For as long as we have birthed life, we have also birthed death. What you feel has been felt since time immemorial, and it has been felt by many, though womb loss is still not widely known or acknowledged. Consider that even in the most optimal conditions, there is only a 30 to 40 percent chance that a clinically recognized pregnancy will occur in a given menstrual cycle, and only about 30 percent of conceived pregnancies progress to live birth.[1] Globally, approximately one in four pregnancies end in miscarriage and 2.6 million pregnancies end in stillbirth.[2] In 2022, 2.3 million newborns died in the first month of life,[3] and approximately 73 million induced abortions occur every year.[4] Womb loss in and after pregnancy is, in fact, a common and regular occurrence, though many of us may struggle with feelings of inadequacy and shame as if such loss is atypical and we are deserving of blame. The prevailing stigma surrounding womb loss makes enduring it all the more challenging as we may feel reluctant to reach out for support and hold on to harmful ideas about our worth. You are not alone, nor are you any less precious and deserving of support.

You are not alone as the anguish of womb loss has been felt, is being felt at this very moment, and will continue to be felt the world over.

Before we go any further, let us reconnect with our breath. It can be hard to breathe if you've recently learned about your womb loss or impending loss and feel pressure to make decisions right away. Or if you have learned of the potential for a loss and have to endure a waiting period before you know for certain. It can be hard to breathe even as you process a loss long since passed. The following practice is an invitation to make the resilient choice to slow down and allow yourself a moment to breathe. So that you can feel grounded. So that you can have the capacity to be present to your grief. So that you can tend to your needs.

GROUNDING BREATHING PRACTICE

Three Deep Breaths

This offering is a simple and short breathing practice. Because you deserve breathing room, and because there is power in the pause. In that fleeting moment between what was and what can be, if you can breathe deeply and connect with your body, you may find yourself more able to understand what you feel and then what you need. Allow yourself this pause so you can make a more intentional decision about what comes next.

The Invitation

When you are ready, take three deep breaths at your own pace and in your own way. You might inhale and exhale through the nose or inhale through the nose and exhale audibly through the mouth. You might close your eyes or soften your gaze as you do so, allowing your awareness to gently follow each breath, letting everything else fade to the background. You might even think the following words as you breathe, allowing them to help you feel grounded in this moment.

Inhale. Exhale. One.
Inhale. Exhale. Two.
Inhale. Exhale. Three.

Your body may want to continue breathing this way, or it may feel like this was enough. Honor what feels right for you.

Sometimes breathing is the most we can bring ourselves to do, the best we can do, when our whole being is overcome. Deciding what comes next may feel like too much to ask of ourselves. If so, breathe, and trust that it is enough for this moment.

A Unique Type of Loss

Womb loss is a type of loss that is as universal as it is unique. It is universal in how common and widespread it is. And it is unique given how intimately it is tied to our own body—the death occurring within our body or, in the case of infant loss, soon after our baby has left our womb. Depending on where you live and the reproductive health care available, you may need to continue your pregnancy or choose to do so until it ends on its own. To carry a dead embryo or fetus inside your body or go days, weeks, or even months knowing that what is growing within you will not survive can be particularly distressing. Thinking back to the two weeks I knowingly carried one of my dead babies inside my body, it is difficult to put into words the sensations and complex feelings I experienced. A part of me wanted to hold on to my baby while another part of me was disturbed that my dead baby was inside me.

And unbeknownst to most, you will eventually need to give birth vaginally or through one of several procedures depending on gestational age, clinical history, personal preference, and access to health care: manual vacuum aspiration (MVA), electric vacuum aspiration (EVA or often clinically referred to as a suction D&C), dilation and evacuation (D&E), dilation and extraction (D&X), or a cesarean section (often referred to as a C-section and less common in the case of pregnancy loss). As with pregnancy and birth in an uncomplicated pregnancy, pregnancy and birth in the context of womb loss can be an intense physical, mental, emotional, and even fatal process for the one birthing. This deeply tactile and intimate type of death, where a part of your body literally dies, where you have to give birth to release from your body what has died or will die, and where your own health is at direct risk, begets a unique type of grief and unique postpartum needs—all of which deserve to be recognized and honored.

When we first learn about our womb loss, we can feel utterly overcome. With shock. With tears. With grief. Experiencing a loss as embodied as ours can make it hard to function, to take in information, to make decisions, to act, or to rest. The following practice is an invitation to help you feel anchored in the present moment so that you have the capacity to tend to what needs your attention.

GROUNDING MINDFULNESS PRACTICE

Choosing an Anchor

When we learn about our womb loss, we may find our thoughts racing as we try hard to make sense of a situation that may have no clear explanation or as we consider options and possibilities beyond those in front of us. Even if time has passed since our loss, our mind may still be overwhelmed by thoughts of it and what could have or should have been. In such situations, we can invite our mind to slow down and even rest by focusing on the moment at hand.

The Invitation

Allow yourself to find a comfortable resting position. Then, as your breath flows in and out naturally, use your senses to make observations of the space around you—perhaps with a simple acknowledgment, either silently or aloud.

This may include sight. Notice where you are and allow your gaze to move slowly around the space. If indoors, you might note things such as a window, table, door, or phone. If outdoors, you might notice trees, clouds, people, or animals.

This may include sound. Notice the sounds coming from you or from your environment. You might note things like the sound of your body breathing, a dog barking, cars driving, people talking.

This may include smell. Notice aromas or maybe the lack thereof. You might note the scent of a candle burning, food cooking, or salty air coming from the sea.

This may include touch. Notice the textures, the weight, or even the temperature of the objects around you or on you. You might note the feel of this book in your hands.

This may include taste. Notice flavors, especially if you've recently had any food or drink, or if there is something in front of you to taste.

Next, choose an anchor among the things you identified. Something that helps you feel grounded. This might be an object you can rest your gaze on, an item you can hold, or an ever-present sound or scent. An anchor can also be another person. You may feel grounded gazing into their eyes or feeling the warmth of their hand in yours. Whatever calls to you, allow it to be a centering force, and know that this is a practice you can return to at any time, especially in moments of struggle.

A Simpler Invitation

If you would like a simpler version of this practice, use your senses to notice just three things around you, naming them either silently or aloud. Then, as you are ready, choose an anchor among those three.

How We Learn About Our Loss

How we learn about our loss can leave as deep and lasting of an impression as the loss itself. Depending on how we feel about the pregnancy, this can be such a deeply heartbreaking moment, and yet those around us may not speak or act in ways that reflect this. It is a moment that demands reverence, but all too often I hear stories from womb loss survivors that speak to an urgent need for our health-care providers, the programs that train them, and the institutions where we receive care to be better equipped to offer grief and trauma-sensitive care. We need and deserve compassionate holding environments so that the trauma of our loss is not compounded by trauma from *how* we learned about it. For example, how might our experiences be if those we trust to support us were to enter and exit the room with reverence, much like entering a breathtaking place in nature or a sacred place of worship? Quietly. Calmly.

With careful steps. Ready to speak with solemnity. We are still in the beginnings of integrating grief and trauma sensitivity into standard pre- and postnatal care, but we can certainly encourage the shifts we want to see so that we and those who follow can receive respectful care that dignifies our loss. And we can begin by reflecting on our own experience of this threshold moment of learning about our loss.

The following practice is an invitation to consider the moment you learned about your womb loss and what you would change. Knowing this may help you advocate for what you need in the future and also help you know what lived wisdom to pass on to others.

What Would You Change?

For this practice, you will need paper and something to write with.

The Invitation

Begin by finding your way into a comfortable position, and as you settle in, allow your awareness to follow your breath as you inhale and as you exhale. When you are ready, begin to think back to the moment when you first learned about your womb loss, to that moment when you learned that your pregnancy would no longer proceed as planned. This moment can look so many ways. For example, this may be when you birthed your loss unexpectedly, when you were told in an appointment that there was no longer a heartbeat, or when you received a heartbreaking diagnosis. If you have experienced more than one known womb loss, you might choose one memory for now and return to the others at a later time, or you might think back to all of those moments as a whole. As you return to that threshold when you transitioned from expectant parent to bereaved parent, begin to consider what you would change about how that moment unfolded. What could have happened differently to make that moment a little more bearable? What would you change so that the part of you who lived that moment could have felt seen, heard, and cared for?

You can share what comes to mind in writing or drawings on your paper. Maybe you feel an intuitive pull to write a letter to the person who confirmed the news, or perhaps write a letter to the you who endured that moment. If, instead, you want to do this reflection practice verbally, consider recording a voice note on your phone. Honor what feels right for you in this moment.

Warming Ginger Tea Recipe

Allow Mother Nature to hold you with this warming, nourishing tea as you begin to process the news of your loss (or impending loss) or reflect back to that time. This simple and universal recipe honors the healing power of ginger. An ancient herbal remedy in many healing traditions, ginger is lauded for its ability to support digestion, ease nausea, strengthen the immune system, and reduce pain, including menstrual cramps.

Whether you are in the midst of your womb loss experience or have already birthed your loss, the act of preparing this tea can be a way to help you feel grounded amidst shock, overwhelm, or other big feelings. It can give your hands something to do while your mind tries to reconcile what you wanted and what is actually unfolding or has unfolded. It can give your mind a break from thinking of what may have been done differently or what may or may not come next as it focuses instead on each step of this recipe. Ginger invites you to slow down and take time for self-tending. Preparing this simple tea can even become a ritual that you come home to through the weeks, months, and years ahead.

- 1-inch-long chunk of fresh ginger peeled and sliced
- 4 cups water
- Honey (or other sweetener) to taste

Connect with the solace Mother Nature has to offer as you notice how the fresh ginger looks, smells, and feels in your hand as you peel and slice it. Take a moment to honor the spirit of this sacred plant and the healing energy it has to share with you. You might consider all that needed to happen for this special plant to come into being and arrive to you and this moment. How it was nurtured by sun, earth, and water before being harvested by human hands and traveling to you.

Add the ginger slices and water to a pot and bring to a boil over high heat. Reduce heat to gently simmer for 5 to 10 minutes, depending on how strongly you would like it to taste. Pour directly into a mug, allowing some ginger slices if desired. Add honey to taste (or other sweetener of choice) and enjoy hot. Allow leftover tea to cool to room temperature before covering and storing in the fridge for up to 4 days. Alternatively, and for ease, you can simply add hot water and a ginger tea bag to a mug, cover, and steep for 5 to 10 minutes.

Contextualizing Womb Loss

Womb loss often comes as a huge surprise, and most of us feel ill-prepared to endure it. Considering the context we experience it in can help us understand why. In a grief-avoidant culture like that of the US, we don't talk openly about death and grief, let alone womb loss (though this is certainly shifting). There is also a prevailing assumption that pregnancy ends with taking home a baby who continues to live beyond infancy. Additionally, how to offer grief and trauma-sensitive care in cases of pregnancy and infant loss is not commonly woven into the standard education, training, and protocols of the health-care providers and birth workers we turn to for support. Any professional training to learn how to work sensitively with bereaved families is typically something that needs to be sought out independently. It makes sense then that womb loss feels like such a shock and that we are unsure how to cope. We don't expect it, and when it happens, our providers often don't know how to support us. Also, depending on where you live, your options for care may be limited, adding another layer of difficulty and grief to an already challenging time.

When your pain is compounded by the context in which you are experiencing womb loss, it can be harder to cope. The following practice is an invitation to pause and simply be. Be present for yourself—for your body, your needs, your grief—in the way you would want others to be. If you are in the midst of your loss, it may be especially challenging to pause and rest. Decisions may need to be made. Research to make those decisions may need to be done. And big feelings may make it hard to do either. If it has been some time since your womb loss, allow yourself to pause and rest now for all the times when it was hard to do so. Wherever you are in your journey, rest can give you strength for what is ahead.

GROUNDING EMBODIMENT PRACTICE

Restorative Side-Lying Pose

After learning about our loss or reflecting back to that time, we need a soft place to land, a place that feels safe to rest so that our bodies can process the memories, information, and feelings that arise. May this practice offer that for you, dear reader.

You will need the following:

- Yoga mat
- 3–4 blankets
- 2 bolsters or pillows
- 1 towel (optional)

The Invitation

When you can have at least 15 minutes of uninterrupted time, find a quiet place where you feel safe resting. You might consider letting people around you know that you need this much time to yourself so they can respect the protective boundary you are establishing. You might feel more at ease tending to your body knowing you've stated your needs. In this embodiment practice, we will be using props to help us ease into a restorative yoga pose and rest. The props are here to hold you so your body does not have to make any effort.

1. When you are ready, create a soft place to land and rest by placing a yoga mat on the floor (if you don't have a yoga mat, find a rug or carpet or simply use blankets), a blanket over it, and a folded blanket

at one end. Place the rest of your props within reach before coming to a seated position.

2. Lean onto one arm, taking your time to slowly lower yourself so you are lying on your side with your head resting on the folded blanket. Bring a soft bend to the knees and consider adding a folded blanket between your legs so the knees can rest level with your hips.

3. If it feels right for your body, place a bolster or pillow in front of you to rest your top arm on and another bolster or pillow behind your back, which can offer an added felt sense of support. For more comfort, you might place a folded towel under your belly to support any weight there, letting this most tender of parts feel held.

4. Finally, you can choose to drape a blanket over your body, creating a warm cocoon. Allow the gentle weight of the blanket to hold and comfort you. If you have someone helping you into this restorative pose, you might ask them to tuck the edges of the blanket under you to deepen the felt sense of being gently cocooned.

5. Once you feel settled in the pose, allow yourself to simply be and breathe, letting your body feel held by the props. Allow your body, which has or is going through so much transition, to soften as it feels safe to do so. And as you rest here, allow anything that feels hard to bear to flow to the parts of your body touching the ground, then out of your body and into the earth. Trust that Mother Earth can hold you and anything you need to release. Honor what you need by lying down for as long as it feels right for you. You can set a timer to wake yourself or emerge on your own naturally.

6. When you are ready, slowly open your eyes if they are closed, gently wiggle your toes and fingers, inviting subtle movement to your body before pressing into your hands to come to a sitting position. Notice how this practice feels for you and consider integrating it into your daily or weekly rhythm. You might bring each day to a close by resting in this pose. You might return to this pose multiple times a day if that feels right. Honor what your body is calling for.

A Simpler Invitation

If it feels like too much for you to set up this restorative pose as described, that's okay. You can simplify this practice by lying on your side on your bed or couch with a pillow under your head, a pillow behind your back, and a pillow in front of you to hug. Pull a blanket over your body and allow yourself to feel cocooned and held.

When Ours Is an Ambiguous Loss

Pregnancy and infant loss can also feel hard to bear because such loss can seem ambiguous and not widely understood by society as a loss worth grieving. It can be considered an *ambiguous loss*, a term Dr. Pauline Boss created to describe loss that lacks documentation of its permanence.[5] This lack of "proof" can make it harder for others to understand and validate the legitimacy of our loss, and it can even make us question what we feel. This lack of acknowledgment of our loss may add another layer to our grief. For example, if you experienced early pregnancy loss, you may not have gotten an ultrasound before your body released the pregnancy. There may be no physical evidence to confirm you were once pregnant, nothing to prove your status as a parent. You may then question whether you can call yourself a mother, a parent, and whether holidays like Mother's Day apply to you. But even if we experience loss later in pregnancy or give birth to a living infant who later dies—when we have more tangible evidence of our loss such as ultrasounds or a more fully formed fetus—it may still feel like society is unsure how to receive us and our grief. And it can be hard to value our own loss if we don't see it modeled around us or affirmed for us. Know that what matters most is what your pregnancy and womb loss mean to you. If you feel grief for your womb loss, then honor that, and know your loss is real and your grief is valid.

The following practice is an invitation to connect with your spirit—what I define as the innate sacred essence of life within you—through ritual. Ritual can be understood as a physical act done with careful attention and loving intention—a reverent pause that allows our spirit to step forward and guide us. Ritual can support us in and through threshold moments, such as when we learn about our womb loss or the potential for it. Ritual can tenderly hold us as we brace ourselves for the worst even as we hope for the best. It does this by connecting us to our spirit, which offers a grounding force that centers us.

The Lighting of a Candle

The ritual of lighting a candle is as simple as it is ancient. Lighting a candle can mark beginnings, and it can mark endings. It can mark major thresholds and smaller transitions. It can be part of a larger ceremony, or it can be a ceremony unto itself.

Even a single candle has the power to shift the energy in a space, in a moment, in a body. It has the power to soften. To slow. To instill a sense of reverence. And it is in this aura of reverence that a candle can bear witness to your spirit and hold space for all that you are, the terrain you have crossed, and all that you carry. You will need a candle and a match or a lighter.

The act of choosing a candle can be infused with as much or as little intention as you want. Consider choosing a candle you love, one with a scent that speaks to you or one in a vessel that draws you in. You might use a candle that was gifted to you and infused with the love from another. Or simply use any candle you find in your home. There is no right or wrong way here. There is only *your* way.

The Invitation

Take a moment to find a quiet and safe place and a comfortable position either standing or seated, with your materials on a flat surface in front of you, be it a bedside table, a remembrance table or altar, or your bathroom counter.

1. Begin by taking a deep, cleansing breath, maybe closing your eyes for a moment or softening your gaze.

2. Then, taking your time, light your candle, allowing for an intention or a prayer to accompany the act if that feels resonant for you. For example, in the spirit of centering you and your needs, you might light your candle while saying silently or aloud: *I am here with my* _____.

Add any feeling words that resonate with you as you cross the threshold from being pregnant to no longer being pregnant—whether for the first time or for another time, or as you reflect back to that time. For example, *I am here with my pain. I am here with my anguish. I am here with my regrets. I am here with my longings.*

3. And breathe. Simply be with your candle, knowing that your candle and the ancient, sacred essence of fire is here to witness you. You might allow your gaze to rest on the soft glow of the flame. You might notice the scent diffusing through the space. You might touch the vessel it is resting in. Stay here for as long as it feels right for you. Allow yourself time. Allow yourself space. And in that time and space, you might notice any thoughts or physical sensations that arise in your body. You might let yourself cry if you feel the urge to do so.

4. When you are ready to bring this practice to a close, I invite you to take a deep breath and blow out your candle, perhaps allowing anything you want to release to follow the smoke as it drifts upward.

You can integrate the lighting of candles into your grieving and post-partum healing process in any way that feels meaningful to you. Make this practice your own, knowing there is no right or wrong way to do it. You can make this ritual a daily practice, a weekly practice, or one you return to whenever you feel called to it.

~

For me, lighting a candle is a cherished nighttime ritual. When the house is finally quiet after the busyness of my family's days, I escape into my bathroom where I turn on a hot shower and light a single candle. There is something instantly and incredibly comforting about showering in this setting, feeling the embrace of hot water as I am cocooned in a soothing darkness with only the company of soft candlelight. It feels womblike. It feels like home.

My thoughts slow. My mind quiets. And I tend to my needs at my pace. Unrushed. Uninterrupted. An incredible feat, truly, after tending to other people and other things all day. In this moment, there is just me, and I savor the peaceful solitude. And in my self-tending, I am grieving and I am healing.

Thank you, sacred Water, I silently say as I turn off the shower.

Thank you, sacred Fire, I silently say as I blow out the candle.

May you, too, find moments to tend to your needs. It is hard, I know. *And* it can be done. Maybe not as regularly as we would want. Maybe not as easily as we would hope. But it can be done, even if it is just for one moment in your day or a moment in your night. It is but a moment, but it is *your* moment.

When Ours Is a Recurrent Loss

If you have experienced womb loss before, my heart goes out to you for all the times you have crossed this threshold of learning of a loss. In the US, recurrent pregnancy loss (RPL) refers to two or more consecutive pregnancy losses that end involuntarily before twenty weeks.[6] For the purposes of this book, however, I would like to honor all who have experienced any form of womb loss more than once. Each pregnancy that ends in loss is a valid loss, and for those who feel grief, know that it is worthy of being grieved and mourned. When you experience womb loss multiple times, each loss can compound the grief of the one(s) that came before, intensifying feelings and adding layers to your grieving and healing process. Each loss can strain your relationship with your body, your partner, and your finances (especially for those who endure fertility treatment, investigational therapies, or overwhelming medical bills).

According to Dr. Atena Asiaii, who specializes in supporting those who experience unexplained infertility and RPL at the Freyja Clinic in California: "Since standard treatment options for recurrent pregnancy loss are limited, people may look into alternative, experimental, and investigational treatments, which can feel very isolating, confusing, and unfamiliar. Finding health-care providers who are knowledgeable and comfortable with these other treatment options is very difficult, adding to the feeling of hopelessness and despair that many who have been through recurrent pregnancy loss already feel."[7] There are many of us who feel the pain of recurrent loss and all the losses associated with it. Know that you are not alone in this.

The following practice is an invitation to ask for what you need. Whether you have experienced womb loss once or many times over, being able to slow down and take time for yourself is an essential skill of resilience. And we all need resilience as we endure.

GROUNDING RELATIONAL PRACTICE

Asking for a Moment

The Invitation

It's okay to ask for time. To ask for space. Asking for a moment to yourself is a way to access your agency in situations such as womb loss that may feel largely out of your control. And it is a way to slow things down and give yourself time to reconnect with your body and its needs.

Practice asking for a moment alone—or rather, letting the other person know you need a moment to yourself. This may be with a partner, family members, or friends. If you are in the midst of your experience of womb loss, you might ask this of your health-care providers, a funeral director, or your employer. You might need a few minutes alone. You might need more. You might use the phrases below, or you might come up with your own.

- I need a moment.
- I need a moment to myself.
- I need time to sit with what you said. Can you come back in a few minutes?

If you have living children, you can model coping skills they can add to their toolbox by showing them that big feelings are okay to feel and sometimes we need some time alone to do that. You might say one of the following or use your own words to let them know you need time to yourself. If you feel you have the capacity to spend time with them later, you can share that too, along with clear instructions so they know what to expect.

- I need some alone time right now.

- I need some alone time right now, but I can join you in _____ minutes. I'll set the timer on my phone, and when it beeps, you can come get me.

- I have big feelings right now and need some alone time, okay? I will open my door when I'm ready to join you.

The asking is simple, but it may not be easy. Especially if you were raised to prioritize others' needs before your own, to make yourself smaller to help others feel comfortable, or to be wary of inconveniencing others. If such things are part of your lived experience, this practice may involve a deep unlearning of these internalized messages. It may be a process to learn to center yourself and your needs. It's okay if it doesn't come naturally. It's okay if it feels uncomfortable. It's okay if it takes time.

Offering from the Collective

The following is an offering from a healing arts practitioner and birth worker I have long admired. Yiska exudes a warmth of spirit that can instantly uplift you, and her understanding and respect for the power of healing touch runs deep. As you will read in her words to follow, offering yourself gentle touch can be potent medicine to soothe your body and your heart when you first learn about your loss, when you think back to that moment, and at any point in your grieving and healing journey. But where you apply touch is important. Whereas existing pregnancy and infant loss resources commonly direct you to place your hands on your womb, such as in meditation, this may be too much too soon. Your womb space may feel incredibly tender—physically and emotionally—and it may take time for you to feel comfortable placing your hands there, if ever. And that's okay. It is for this reason that I have included Yiska's offering here, in chapter 1, so that you have a tool for self-tending that utilizes touch without touching your womb.

Self-Havening Touch

What it is

Havening is a powerful healing modality that uses soothing downward strokes applied to the hands, arms, and face to increase slow brain wave activity, which has been shown to relieve the effects of stored trauma, fear, anxiety, and other emotional stresses. While Havening Touch can be offered in a therapeutic context by a trained Havening practitioner, self-havening touch can be practiced by anyone, at any time, with positive stand-alone effects.

How it can support you

The power of touch to provide comfort is well known. Comforting touch can help lower stress hormone levels and increase the presence of biochemicals such as serotonin, dopamine, endorphins, and oxytocin, which are associated with our capacity to feel satisfied, peaceful, connected, and loved. Touch is often just the right "remedy" for the feelings of aloneness and disconnection so common to the experience of womb loss.

When healing touch is recommended for those who've experienced womb loss, people may be directed to bring hands to their womb space, which may feel good for some, but for others this can feel overwhelming, too painful, or too soon. To experience the comfort of touch in a less direct way can make it feel more accessible. This kind of touch can also be combined with other forms of meditation or visualization you may already be using to help your body, mind, and spirit process your loss.

Self-havening touch is something I used to comfort myself through my own grief and experiences of loss. I offered myself this touch in quiet moments of silence, in moments of wailing and sobbing, even in moments of anger at life or myself. I offered myself this touch as a way to tend my heart through those painful chapters, not to take the feelings away but to help me feel cared for and held while I felt the truths of my heart in any given moment, whatever needed to be felt. It always left me feeling calmer and quieter on the other side.

Self-Havening Touch to Gently Honor Grief

A self-tending practice

Before I describe the practice, keep in mind that it is always okay if this is not what you need at this moment in your grieving process. Take this as a simple invitation or an experiment to discover if the power of self-soothing touch is something that can help support you at this moment in time.

Self-havening can be done anywhere, anytime, even during a shower, although typically you would start by doing this practice in a comfortable seat. Beginning with your arms and hands in the shape of a self-hug, you'll start by stroking your arms downward, from your shoulders to your elbows. Repeat this motion at a pace that feels good, with an amount of pressure that feels right to you, neither too firm nor too light.

After a few moments, if you haven't already closed your eyes, try turning your gaze inward and allow yourself to feel. To cry and release if that is what's there. Perhaps you will simply take this time to pause and breathe, focusing on your inhalation and exhalation. Grief can sometimes take our breath away, and this can be a moment to take it back, to see if a deeper breath is available. Take this moment to simply be in your pain or your acceptance. Your gratitude, your anger. Your fear, your despair, your hope. Use this moment to give yourself space to be where you are without distraction, with your full attention and care. Your nervous system will thank you.

I recommend making space for five minutes of this self-havening touch to start. I typically self-haven for five to twenty minutes daily. You are welcome to do more or less once you become familiar with the effects of this practice in your body. If your hands feel drawn to bring your self-havening touch to your belly and womb, that is also welcome. This same Havening Touch can also be applied to your face with repeated downward strokes from forehead down your cheeks, and by rubbing your hands together. Petting an animal can have similar effects.

In the end, comforting touch is just one of many ways to honor your loss, your body, your feelings, and your heart. It's a powerful one I hope you will explore to support your womb and heart healing.

A Gentle Closing

Thank you for being here. For showing up for yourself, your body, and your grief as we explored the threshold moment of learning about your womb loss. This time in your fertility journey is one worth reflecting on as it so often leaves deep impressions that we may or may not be aware of. Impressions that may be influencing how we show up in our lives. Impressions that may be in need of tending even many years later. Whether you are newly bereaved or reflecting back to this threshold, may you be gentle with yourself. Know that you are not alone, that there is support within these pages and beyond. And know that it's okay to cry. As much as you need to. For as long as you need to.

As this chapter comes to a close, I invite you to pause for a few breaths and with the closing verse to help you transition gently back into your life or to the next part of the book. And if anything in this chapter activated a strong response, consider doing something more to feel grounded. This may be an act of self-tending or reaching out to someone you trust for support. Honor what you need in this moment.

I am here, as I am.
And so it is.

You are here.
And we are with you.

CHAPTER 2

Birthing Your Loss

What is your body calling for in this moment?

There are moments that stand out in my memory of birthing my first pregnancy loss. The soft glow of the afternoon sunlight filtering into the darkness of the bathroom, the door left slightly ajar. How soothing both the darkness and the natural light felt. Witnessing myself in a very primal moment as I sat naked, with legs set wide, hands holding on to the edges of the toilet seat as the contractions intensified—and how this realization washed over me leaving me shocked: *I'm giving birth.* Moments later, this thought emerged: *My body knows how to do this.*

I had given birth once before—vaginally without medication—and I knew there was a purpose to the pain, that the contractions were my body's way of moving my baby down and out. Experience had taught me that I could endure the contractions by breathing deeply, and if I followed my body's cues, it would guide me into positions that would help my womb release what it carried. As I reassured myself, I felt my physical body soften and a sense of calm arise. In that state, I was able to listen more easily to what my body was calling for, which was to be in a warm shower alternating between a fetal position and being on hands and knees, letting the water console me.

~

I wish my doctor had told me that releasing an early pregnancy loss meant I was essentially giving birth. Knowing this, I could have mentally prepared myself for labor, not just bleeding. For contractions, not just cramping. At the same time, I appreciate how I was able to pull from my own internal source of resilience and trust my body's lived wisdom. Know, dear reader, that you can too. I did the best I could that day. And truly, that is all any of us can do.

You Too Give Birth

Once you are pregnant, what is growing within you will eventually need to leave your body no matter the length of gestation, whether an embryo developed or not, or whether the embryo, fetus, or baby is living or has already died in utero (in your womb). The word *birth* simply means "*to bring forth.*"[1]

Anyone who is pregnant will eventually release the pregnancy, and reframing it as birth can help afford greater regard for a process that can be so momentous and so physically, mentally, and emotionally demanding. In the context of pregnancy and infant loss, you may experience a first trimester birth, a second trimester birth, or a third trimester birth. Some may labor and deliver vaginally without intervention. Some may labor, get an epidural, and deliver vaginally. Others may go from being pregnant to not being pregnant without feeling a single contraction through the course of a procedure. No matter when or how, know that you have given birth or will give birth, even if you do not have a living baby to hold. Reframing it this way can also help clarify and instill the truth that you are or will be postpartum after pregnancy and infant loss. You were or are pregnant, you have or will give birth, and you are or will be postpartum. The process is the same whether or not our pregnancy ends with a living child. And if the word *birth* and the idea of giving birth do not resonate with you, that is okay too. You get to choose how to name your experiences.

The following practice is an invitation to explore breathing while gently lengthening the exhalation, which can signal to your body that all is well and you can relax. If you are preparing for the physical release of your loss, deep breathing with intentional longer exhalations can help you bear painful waves of contractions by encouraging your body to soften rather than tense up. It can also help you feel grounded before, during (if you are awake), and after a procedure. If your body has already released your pregnancy, you can turn to this and other breathing practices whenever you want to feel more grounded, whenever your grief feels overwhelming, or whenever your postbirth body wants to feel more at ease, even if just for a moment.

Candle Breathing

Your breath is a powerful tool that you can access anytime, anywhere, for valuable self-tending. Visualizing a candle can be grounding as it allows your mind to focus on a single thing. And in this practice, the act of blowing out a candle with a long exhalation can help your body soften by activating your parasympathetic nervous system, which tells your body you are safe and can rest.

The Invitation

As you are ready, begin by deepening your breath and either closing your eyes or softening your gaze. Allow your awareness to follow each inhalation and each exhalation. Then, taking your time, imagine a candle in your mind's eye, its flame casting a warm glow. Picturing this, inhale through the nose then exhale through the mouth, as if you were trying to gently blow out the flame with a long exhalation, much like blowing out birthday candles. You might also make your exhalation audible and allow your mind to focus on the sound. Continue breathing in this way for a few more breaths or for however long it feels right for you. When you feel ready to bring this breathing practice to a close, return to your normal breath while pressing down through the parts of you resting on the earth. Then, taking your time, slowly open your eyes if they are closed.

If it feels uncomfortable to extend your exhalation, you might consider taking just three (or more) deep breaths as described in chapter 1. Figuring out which embodied practices work best for you is a process. Please honor what feels safe and right in your body, keeping in mind that your preferences may shift over time.

The Care You Deserve

It is important to consider factors that influence the quality of care you receive as you prepare for birth or the quality of care you received if you are reflecting back to this time. This includes how beliefs about race and gender shape our laws, policies, hospital practices, and the training health-care providers receive. *Gender bias* is a term often used to describe how women are widely and routinely dismissed and not taken seriously when expressing concerns about their health, including their pregnancies, and are often thought to be exaggerating their pain.[2] This can lead to a delay in diagnoses, inadequate symptom relief, and death not only among pregnant women but transgender and nonbinary pregnant people too.[3] Women of color face the added factor of racial bias, with Black, American Indian and Alaska Native (AIAN) women experiencing higher rates of pregnancy-related death than White women, especially during the COVID-19 pandemic.[4] Black, AIAN, and Native Hawaiian and Other Pacific Islander (NHOPI) women also experience pregnancies ending in higher infant mortality rates than White women.[4] Quite counter to the way our culture primarily regards pregnancy as a time of celebration is the truth that pregnancy can be deadly, and those who survive it deserve the utmost support and respect.

As you endure womb loss within systems that are not necessarily designed to tend to our needs with compassion, know that you deserve respectful, quality health care that is unbiased and trauma-free. You deserve to work with providers who help you feel seen, listened to, and cared for; this includes being open to and understanding with your questions and concerns. You deserve to receive health care that validates your loss as real, your grief as valid, and sees to your needs with sensitivity and reverence. And while it can be incredibly hard to advocate for yourself in the midst of or even after womb loss, know that you can. You can use your voice to state your needs. You can use your voice to ask others to help you get your needs met. You can also look for providers who can meet your needs by searching on the internet; asking friends, family, and other providers for referrals; and connecting with organizations specifically dedicated to supporting survivors of pregnancy and infant loss such as those listed in the resources section at the end of this book.

The following practice is an invitation to nurture the connection between your mind and body so that it may become easier to notice your body's cues and understand what it is trying to tell you through sensations. Our bodies and our intuition will tell us if something is wrong, if something needs our attention, if something needs to change so we can feel safe. Listen to what your body is telling you, and if it's saying you deserve better, have courage to advocate for yourself.

GROUNDING MINDFULNESS PRACTICE

A Gentle Body Scan

This mindfulness practice invites you to do a light body scan, noting any sensations as you go. It is an invitation to be a companion to yourself. To bear witness to your body and what is present for you, in you, with a soft, gentle awareness. To practice listening to what it has to say.

The Invitation

1. As you feel ready, find a comfortable resting position either seated or lying down. Then, taking your time, begin by inviting your awareness to your scalp and face, noting any sensations here with gentleness. Simply notice without trying to change anything.

2. Allow your awareness to flow down into your neck and shoulders, noting what is present in these areas of your body. Again, with gentleness and without trying to change anything. When you are ready, invite your awareness down into your arms, hands, and fingers, noting any sensations before drawing your awareness up into your chest. Gently notice what is present for you here.

3. Next, allow your awareness to carefully flow down to your belly, your womb space. This is a deeply tender place, so if your instinct is to avoid this part of you, that is completely understandable and okay. When you are ready, bring your awareness into your back body: your upper back, middle back, low back, and glutes. Notice any sensations here with gentleness. Taking your time, allow your awareness to flow into your hips,

Birthing Your Loss   47

noting any sensations. Be extra gentle with yourself here as the hips are known to hold unprocessed emotions, memories, trauma. This is why you might find yourself crying after doing hip-opening poses in yoga.

4. Finally, allow your awareness to flow into your legs, feet, and toes, noting any sensations with gentleness as you make your way down the body.

5. To bring this practice to a close, take a few deep breaths before gently wiggling your fingers and toes to invite movement back into your body.

This is a practice you can turn to whenever you need support. Whenever the mind has trouble quieting. Whenever the next step isn't clear. Whenever the next step is hard to bear.

Notice and breathe.
Notice and breathe.
Notice and breathe.

Notice and breathe, and let this be enough as you do your best to endure.

Options for Care

Birthing your loss can be incredibly challenging mentally, emotionally, and physically. Most of us who birth loss do so in a culture that does not prepare us for this kind of birth outcome. We may know what to expect from births that proceed safely and result in living children who continue to live, but many of us only come to learn the details of birthing loss through personal experience. Knowing what to expect and what options exist can help you endure this part of your womb loss experience with a little less fear and anxiety.

Generally, there are three options for birthing loss: expectant management (allowing your body to release the pregnancy on its own without intervention), medical management (use of medication to support the body in releasing the pregnancy), and procedural management (use of a procedure(s) to remove the pregnancy). At times, treatment options are combined. For example, in an early pregnancy loss, you may choose to give your body time to go into labor naturally (expectant management), but later decide to take medication to initiate labor (medical management), and then need to have a procedure to remove retained uterine tissue (procedural management). If you are preparing to birth your loss, the following is a brief overview of options that are typically available. Your options for care depend on many factors, including the circumstances of your particular form of womb loss, where you live, what reproductive health care is available, and cost. It is important to talk to your health-care provider to learn:

- What options are appropriate for you
- What happens and what you might expect to feel
- What risks are involved (including impact on future fertility)
- What recovery typically looks like (duration and what you can and cannot do during that time)
- What happens to the pregnancy tissue, to your baby, after you give birth (including options for genetic testing of the pregnancy tissue)
- What the cost for treatment is and how much will you be responsible for

Options for First Trimester Pregnancy Loss

1. Allow your body to go into labor on its own and birth vaginally (expectant management).

2. Still allow your body to birth vaginally but with the support of medication to induce labor (medical management).

3. Use a procedure called manual vacuum aspiration (MVA) or electric vacuum aspiration (EVA or suction D&C) to remove the pregnancy directly from the womb (procedural management). Sharp curettage is no longer recommended.

Options for Second Trimester Pregnancy Loss

1. Be admitted to a hospital to have labor induced and birth vaginally (medical management also referred to as labor induction).

2. Use a procedure called dilation and evacuation (D&E) or dilation and extraction (D&X) to remove the pregnancy directly from the womb (procedural management).

Options for Third Trimester Pregnancy Loss

1. Allow your body to go into labor on its own and then go to the hospital for vaginal delivery (expectant management).

2. Be admitted to a hospital to have labor induced and birth vaginally (labor induction).

3. Proceed with cesarean section (used in select circumstances).

Note that in the case of ectopic pregnancy (when a fertilized egg implants outside of the uterus), which is a very dangerous form of a nonviable pregnancy that can result in fallopian tube rupture, treatment options vary from those listed above. Options for treating ectopic pregnancy typically include expectant management, where the pregnancy is simply monitored if it is expected to resolve on its own, or more commonly, the use of medication to stop the growth of cells or a procedure to either remove the pregnancy from the tube or to remove the whole fallopian tube.

Also worth noting is that delivery by C-section, which is major surgery, is not usually an option if the fetus is no longer alive in the womb. At that point, since the focus is now solely on your safety, labor and vaginal delivery is a safer option. Dr. Kate White, author of *Your Guide to Miscarriage & Pregnancy Loss: Hope and Healing When You're No Longer Expecting*, says this on the topic: "I completely understand why the idea of putting you through labor seems cruel when you're not going to have the happy outcome that you wanted. But the C-section was developed as a technique to try to deliver the baby safely during a complicated or dangerous delivery . . . In fact, a C-section has serious immediate and long-term risks to the mother's health."[5] Dr. White is an OB-GYN and miscarriage survivor with a gift for explaining the medical side of womb loss in a way that is easy to understand with sensitivity and warmth. I highly recommend her book as a resource as you explore your options.

If you have yet to give birth, the following practice is an invitation to pause and reflect on what you may want for labor and delivery, for the ending of your pregnancy. If you have already birthed your loss and are reflecting back to that time, perhaps read through the following and consider what you might have done differently knowing what you know now.

GROUNDING REFLECTION PRACTICE

Birth Plan for Womb Loss

For those who are still pregnant and have yet to give birth, consider creating a birth plan—a document that clearly outlines your preferences for three main categories: (1) labor and delivery, (2) care of the pregnancy tissue/your baby's remains, or end of life care if your infant is born alive, and (3) memory making. Even if you choose not to share it with anyone, it can be a helpful process to consider your options and make meaningful choices for the duration of your pregnancy, labor, and birth, and for those who birth living infants, the limited time you have with your baby. You will need paper and something to write with; alternatively, you can note your preferences directly in the book.

The Invitation

Alone, or together with a partner or other support person, create a birth plan for your womb loss. The following are a series of items commonly found on such plans. Please note that your options may vary depending on factors such as the type of womb loss you are experiencing, how far along your pregnancy has progressed, and health care that is available where you live. You can choose to go through these prompts and compile them into one document. You can also choose to do an online search with keywords such as "birth plan for baby loss" or "perinatal palliative birth plan," or ask your health-care provider for guidance and resources. You might also consider hiring a doula who specializes in supporting birth in the context of loss (also known as a bereavement doula or a full-spectrum doula) to help you create the birth plan and remind you of it in labor. If you are partnered, you might change "I" to "we."

Labor and Delivery

- I would/would not like to birth in a bereavement suite if available (special rooms to birth away from the sights and sounds of other births and live babies).

- I would/would not like to be informed of what to expect as the process unfolds to avoid being taken by surprise.

- I would/would not like the presence of a support person dedicated to me and my needs (e.g., partner, parent, birth doula, full-spectrum doula, bereavement doula).

- I would/would not like to have an epidural.

- I would/would not like to learn about other options for pain management and medications during labor and delivery.

- I would/would not like a sign on our door informing staff that we are experiencing pregnancy/infant loss.

- I would/would not like staff to refer to my baby by name. My baby's name is _____.

- I would/would not like our baby's heartbeat monitored during labor.

- If there is a loss of the heartbeat prior to delivery, we do/do not wish to be informed.

- I would/would not like a cesarean section if fetal distress occurs.

- I would like _____ to cut the umbilical cord, if possible.

- I would/would not like to see the remains/my baby, or I am not sure.

- I would/would not like to hold the remains/my baby, or I am not sure.

- I would like the remains/my baby to be handed immediately to me or _____.

- I would like time alone before holding the remains/my baby.

- I would/would not like a ritual (e.g., naming ceremony, blessing, baptism) performed after giving birth.

- I would like the following person to perform a ritual: _____.

- I would/would not like a cooling cot or cooling blanket (these are special cooling devices that preserve the remains/your baby's body so that you can spend more time together).

- I would/would not like students or health-care professionals in training involved in care.

Comfort Measures for Infant Loss (infant born alive)

- Medication (for comfort and to ease pain): Y/N

- Oxygen: Y/N

- Skin-to-skin contact: Y/N

- Oral comfort measures (e.g., pacifiers): Y/N

- Feeding (breast milk, formula, sugar-water): Y/N

- I would/would not like to talk with someone about breastfeeding/ expressing milk.

Connecting to Baby (living or deceased)

- I would/would not like my baby to stay in the room as long as possible.

- I would/would not like to bathe and dress my baby.

- I would/would not like to dress my baby in clothes I have brought.

- I would/would not like help from the nursing staff to bathe and dress my baby.

- I would/would not like support to know how to care for my newborn at home (i.e., for newborns with life-limiting conditions).

Lactation Support After Loss

- I would/would not like to talk with someone about expressing and donating my milk.

- I would/would not like to talk with someone about how to decrease and eventually stop my milk production.

Support for Living Children

- I would/would not like help talking to our living children.

- I would/would not like my living children to meet their sibling(s).
- I would/would not like my living children to be part of memory-making activities.
- I would/would not like resources and recommendations for professionals who can help our living children understand and process the loss.

Memory Making

- I would/would not like pictures of the remains/my baby.
- I would/would not like video of the remains/my baby.
- I would/would not like the following:
  - Crib card/band
  - Birth certificate/death certificate if available
  - Lock of hair
  - Hand/foot mold
  - Other:

Handling of Remains

- I would/would not like support making arrangements for a funeral/memorial service.
- I would/would not like to take the remains/my baby home if possible.
- I would/would not like to receive information about hospital options for sensitive handling of the remains (such as communal cremation).

Additional Testing (to try to determine a cause of condition/death)

- I would/would not like to have blood tests conducted.
- I would/would not like to have X-rays/MRI.
- I would/would not like to have an autopsy.
- I would/would not like to discuss testing options with a physician or genetic counselor.

Red Raspberry Leaf Infusion Recipe

The prospect of giving birth when your baby is already dead inside your body or doing so when you anticipate your baby dying can be beyond words. So tied are we to the idea that giving birth means giving birth to living babies who will continue to live past infancy. And yet all pregnancies must end, and what grows within our wombs must eventually be released. That you will give birth or have given birth to loss may stand in such stark, heartbreaking contrast to what you may have wanted for yourself. For your baby. For your family. I understand this deeply, and so do many others. We are with you as you prepare for birth or as you look back to the birthing of your loss.

Red raspberry leaf (also known as raspberry leaf) is a plant that has been used for centuries to strengthen the womb during pregnancy, induce labor, and shorten the duration of labor. In this simple and universal infusion recipe (an infusion being stronger than tea due to the longer steeping time), we invite red raspberry to support you as you prepare for birth or as you heal your womb after loss. Rich in antioxidants, this plant can also help protect your body from chronic disease and inflammation, and it is said to help ease discomfort related to menstruation.

- 2 tea bags red raspberry leaf
- 1 cinnamon stick
- 32-ounce mason jar
- Honey (or other sweetener) to taste

Add tea bags and cinnamon stick to the mason jar (you can tape the strings of the tea bags to the outside of the jar to keep from falling in) and fill with boiling water. Seal and let sit for at least 4 hours to allow ample time for the plant medicine to be drawn out. Enjoy warm with honey and allow the sensation of warmth to ground you when you notice yourself feeling anxious, overwhelmed, withdrawing, or experiencing other responses that make it difficult to be present for the moment at hand. Drink mindfully, taking note of each aspect of the experience: seeing your hands raise the cup, feeling the sensation of the cup making contact with your lips, noticing how the warm liquid feels as it flows into your body, and noting the flavor lingering on your tongue. As you hold and drink the infusion, allow its warmth to soften your body, soothe your feelings, and quiet your thoughts, even if just for a moment.

Home Birth for Early Pregnancy Loss

Expectant management and medical management of an early pregnancy loss is essentially a home birth. We are commonly told that we will experience cramping and bleeding, but it may help to understand that you are in fact giving birth, that you will feel contractions as your womb releases what it holds inside, and that blood and tissue (which may look like large blood clots and even a noticeable fetus) will be released through your vagina. Reframing it in this way can help you feel more emotionally prepared to cross this tremendous threshold moment from pregnant to no longer pregnant.

You can also ask your health-care provider if they offer support while you birth at home. For example, when I was pregnant after two losses, I asked one of my midwives what the midwifery practice did if a patient experienced pregnancy loss. I was told that the midwives could offer phone support while the patient birthed at home. Knowing this option was available felt reassuring. You might also do an internet search to see if there are any support hotlines in your area. For example, the Doula Project in New York City offers national, 24/7 text support from doulas for those birthing their loss at home with the support of medication. Or you can secure in-person doula support from a birth or full-spectrum doula (a doula who offers support across the spectrum of reproduction including conception, pregnancy, birth, postpartum, and loss); these doulas are non-medical birth workers who can offer emotional support, information, and resources. Doula Vicki Bloom of The Doula Project powerfully describes the role of doulas in the context of loss—that in addition to the same physical comfort measures offered in pregnancies expected to end with living children (e.g., massage, hot pads, and hand-holding), it's also about "holding space for that person, whatever they're feeling, letting them feel in the moment, helping them feel safe, helping them feel like they're having an experience that they need to have in a way that feels comforting to them."[6]

You might also consider if it would be meaningful to have someone take photos or a video of your labor and birth—something to honor your moving through this immense threshold. I once came across a photo series online showing a woman birthing her early pregnancy loss at home with her partner and midwife. The photos were stunning, capturing the vivid reality of pain as the woman labored on the ground on all fours and later in the bathroom on the toilet and then the heartbreaking awe as the couple held and gazed lovingly at their tiny, dead baby.

Reframing the release of an early pregnancy loss as a home birth can also help you prepare for the practical aspects. You might consider preparing the following in addition to doing your own research, keeping in mind that you will likely be met with web pages that assume you are birthing a living child. If you are reflecting back to this time, consider whether reframing this threshold as a birth affects how you view your experience.

- Container with a lid to store the pregnancy tissue for genetic testing (contact your health-care provider to discuss this option), burial at a location of your choice, or burial or cremation through a local funeral home
- Saline solution to clean off and store pregnancy tissue
- Gloves and tweezers to help separate pregnancy tissue from blood clots if collecting pregnancy tissue
- Toilet hat and strainer/colander to catch pregnancy tissue
- Plastic covering underneath old bedsheets for laboring in bed
- Pain-relief medication (talk to your health-care provider to discuss options)
- Heating pad to place on your belly for pain relief
- Water and snacks
- Calming music, essential oils, and candles for a soothing environment
- Highly absorbent maxi pads for postpartum bleeding
- Postpartum mesh underwear
- Loose, comfortable clothing

The following practices invite you to slow down, pause, and be with your body in silence so you may hear what it needs. You can turn to these two yoga poses when laboring to support you as you experience intense sensations that may be new and overwhelming. They are also poses you can find solace in immediately after or long after birth. May they offer you a safe place to land and simply be.

Polar Bear Pose and Child's Pose

It can be hard to honor what our bodies intuitively need when we are in pain, when we we're not taught how to listen to our bodies, when this instinct was not modeled for us, and when we live in cultures that encourage doing over being. If you are preparing to birth your loss, know that you can turn to Polar Bear or Child's Pose to gently stretch your body, cope with pain during labor, and offer yourself quiet moments of grounding so you may hear what your body is trying to tell you. If your body has already released the pregnancy, if you have already birthed your loss, know that you can also turn to these poses to help you hear what your body needs and for a felt experience of being grounded and centered.

You will need the following:

* Yoga mat

* 1 yoga block or a folded blanket

* 1–2 blankets

The Invitation

To begin, create a soft place to land by placing a yoga mat on the ground and a folded blanket(s) on top. If you don't have a yoga mat, that is completely fine. Instead, use blankets or find a soft rug or carpet for this pose. Take your time and move at your own pace as you make your way into a kneeling position, placing the palms of your hands on the earth directly below the shoulders to come into tabletop position. If it feels comfortable in your body, begin to transition from your hands to your forearms, coming into Polar Bear Pose. Perhaps stay here for three breaths, or begin to explore gentle dynamic movement such as slowly rocking forward and backward. Try drawing circles with the hips, moving in one direction and then the other. Notice what sensations arise in your body and honor what feels right for you. You might ask yourself, *What does my body need in this moment?*

If it feels accessible, you can move from Polar Bear to Child's Pose. To do this, set your knees wider than hip distance apart and bring the big toes to touch. Allow your sit bones to move toward your heels as you either stretch your arms forward, resting your palms face up or down, or bring your arms to your sides, allowing your shoulders to melt forward. Rest your forehead or cheek on a block or folded blanket. You might place a rolled blanket directly behind the backs of the knees if this is comfortable while you rest and breathe. Pause here, listen to the sensations in your body, and follow its lead. Rest in stillness, or perhaps explore gentle, dynamic movement such as rocking slowly forward onto hands and knees and back into Child's Pose. Honor what your body needs in this moment.

Labor Pain

If you are releasing your pregnancy through vaginal delivery, whether you are birthing in or out of a hospital, be prepared to tend to the pain of contractions. If you have never experienced labor, contractions may be a shocking and especially challenging experience. Contractions occur when the muscles of your uterus repeatedly tighten then relax, helping to push what is held within your womb out of your body through the vagina. They can feel different for each person and even differ for the same person between pregnancies. Typically, contractions feel like waves of increasingly intense cramping in your belly and low back. As labor progresses, contractions become stronger and occur more frequently with less time in between to rest. They can become so painful that it is difficult to talk or move.

You, too, are giving birth, so consider coping techniques typically recommended for labor and delivery. Perhaps create a soft, soothing space with dim lighting and calming music to settle in for labor. To help ease the pain of contractions, consider applying a heating pad, resting in a warm shower, inhaling the scent of a comforting essential oil, or receiving a gentle massage from your partner or other support person. You might secure the services of a birth doula or full-spectrum doula, or talk to your health-care provider about a short course of stronger pain medication. Listen to your body and follow its urgings. You may intuitively feel like being on the ground, finding your way into Polar Bear or Child's Pose. You may feel like walking around or sitting on the toilet. If you are birthing in a hospital, ask what pain-relief options may be available, such as an epidural, which is a numbing medicine administered through an injection in the low back.

Whether you are preparing for labor and delivery or reflecting back to this time, the following practice is an invitation to center yourself so that you may feel more comfortable doing so when in labor and in your life beyond this threshold moment.

GROUNDING RITUAL PRACTICE

Choose Yourself First: A Morning Practice

Centering your needs is a process, and it can take time and practice to embody the deep knowing that you are worthy of care. May this daily practice of doing something simple for yourself first, before tending to anything or anyone else, nurture your ability to honor your needs.

The Invitation

Choose a simple embodiment practice to start each day this week. This could be taking three deep breaths right when you wake up. It could be doing a yoga pose like Polar Bear or Child's Pose for three breaths when you first get out of bed. This could also be making yourself a warm cup of tea and drinking it mindfully before doing anything else. Whatever it is, let it be simple so it feels doable. And give yourself permission to try different morning rituals until you find one (or more) that feels right for you.

Caring for What Remains

Know that once your body releases the pregnancy, you may see the embryo or fetus in the tissue that you pass. The farther along you are in your pregnancy, the larger and more formed the remains may be. While this may be obvious, many of us are completely shocked to experience it. What you do with the remains, your baby, is a personal decision, though it may also depend on the gestational age of the embryo or fetus and where you give birth. In early pregnancy loss, it is common to labor and birth at home, often on the toilet. If you birth over the toilet, know that you can choose to look into it or not. You can choose to take the pregnancy tissue out of the toilet (you can also place a strainer or container over the toilet seat to catch it), or you can choose to flush it. If you are unsure whether to look down, perhaps ask a partner or support person to do so and describe what they see before you make a decision. If you birth your loss in the shower, you might consider plugging the drain or placing a drain protecter over it to catch the remains. If you choose to keep the remains, you can handle them in a number of ways:

- Preserve the remains in a container in the fridge for testing (contact your health-care provider to discuss this option).

- Bury the remains in a place that is meaningful to you, such as in your backyard or in a planter of flowers.

- Contact a local hospital for sensitive handling of remains, such as communal cremation.

- Contact a local funeral home to explore possible options for cremation, burial, and memorial services.

- If you are birthing in a hospital, ask what options are available for sensitive care of the remains. Your options may include those indicated in the sample birth plan we covered earlier and can depend on factors such as gestational age, the hospital's protocols, and the laws in your region.

The following practices invite you to reach out to your community for support and allow others to tend to you in your time of need. You might think of asking for support as a skill, something that may not come easily at first but can get easier the more you do it. Know that you do not have to cross this threshold of birthing your loss alone.

A Womb Loss Blessing

The Invitation

Consider asking a loved one or other support person like a doula to hold space to honor you, your womb loss, and your baby with a womb loss blessing ceremony. Much like a mother blessing, which is a mother-centered counterpart to a baby shower, a womb loss blessing is a time for you to feel held within a loving circle of support before giving birth to your loss or afterward in your postpartum time. The intention here is to create a space where you feel safe to be vulnerable and an opportunity for you to feel witnessed. Make the ceremony your own so that it feels meaningful and supportive. You and the host can discuss any preferences or desires you have and co-create the ceremony. If you don't have the capacity to plan, that's okay too. You can ask the host to design it, perhaps giving them basic information such as the name of your baby if they have one, the faith tradition you may follow, and a list of names and contact information of the people you would like to invite. It can be an intimate gathering of a few loved ones in someone's home or a beautiful place outside where you can integrate the healing power of nature. The following is a sample outline you can reference as you decide what feels right for you.

Setup: The host can invite everyone to sit in a circle on the ground or in chairs. You can be part of the circle or allow yourself to feel held by sitting or lying in the center, perhaps cocooned in a warm blanket. The host can then say the following or simply use this as a guide for their own words.

If you are still pregnant: *Welcome. Thank you all for coming. We gather here today to hold space for you, [your name], at this tender time as you prepare to give birth/give birth to [name of baby if given one]. Know that you are not alone. We are with you, ready to hold you for as long as you need to be held, and to tend to you for as long as you need tending.*

If you have already given birth: *Welcome. Thank you all for coming. We gather here today to hold space for you, [your name], at this tender time as you*

grieve the end of your pregnancy and endure the postpartum time without your
baby. Know that you are not alone. We are with you, ready to hold you for as
long as you need to be held and tend to you for as long as you need tending.

Ritual: *We will now pass around a candle. You are welcome to hold it and*
share words for [your name], imbuing the candle with your message and energy
of love, so that even after we leave, [your name] can feel our presence and know
[your pronoun] is loved.

Closing: This can be a time for you to share words of your own, dear reader,
or not. It is your choice.

Thank you for coming and helping us to hold [your name] in love. I invite
you to join me in taking three deep breaths to help bring this gathering to a
gentle close.

After: Depending on your capacity, guests may stay after to share food and
drink, offering an opportunity for them to connect with you one-on-one.

GROUNDING RELATIONAL PRACTICE #2

A Community of Candles

The Invitation

Reach out to the people in your support network and ask them to light a candle for you when you are laboring in a symbolic act of support. You might ask
them to light it on the day and time you plan on taking medication to encourage labor at home, you will be induced in the hospital, or you will undergo
your procedure. If you are letting your body release your pregnancy in its own
time, a partner or other support person can let them know when you go into
labor and also be a point of contact for any questions or messages of support.
Knowing that people are pausing and taking a moment to light a candle in your
honor can help you feel the truth that you are not alone in this experience. You
are in fact surrounded by the warmth and love of your people.

Offering from the Collective

The following is an offering from my beloved friend Molly, a Somatic Experiencing® (SE) Practitioner and trauma-informed yoga teacher. We met well over a decade ago as volunteers for a rape crisis center in Chicago, and I have had the honor of watching her start and grow the nonprofit organization *The Breathe Network*, which helps connect survivors of sexual trauma with trauma-informed, holistic healing practitioners. Because of the deeply embodied nature of womb loss, it is essential that we connect with our body in ways that feel safe and manageable. It is also essential that we come to know that our bodies are as much a source of healing as a source of pain. Molly speaks to this with her signature warmth and richness of words and from her own embodied experience of womb loss.

AN OFFERING BY MOLLY BOEDER HARRIS

Somatic Experiencing

What it is

Somatic Experiencing (SE) was created by somatic psychotherapist Dr. Peter Levine as a body-oriented approach for renegotiating trauma and healing the impacts of stress and overwhelm. SE integrates his multidisciplinary studies of stress physiology, ethology, biology, neuroscience, psychology, and Indigenous healing practices. For me, it is also a relational, holistic philosophy on living that recognizes our body as a primary source of healing and a resource we can call upon in our daily lives to nurture and empower ourselves, as well as those around us. Typically, SE sessions are an hour-long meeting, which can happen in person or online. Rather than being a formulaic practice, each session is tailored to the individual's life experiences, the resources they are arriving with, and their intentions for the healing work. It is an organic collaboration as the SE practitioner and participant track five channels of human experience—sensation in the body, imagery, behaviors, emotions, and meaning—and together notice cycles of activation and settling. By moving in an intentionally incremental way, SE aims to reduce the risk of overwhelming the nervous system while simultaneously increasing the possibility for unresolved or incomplete physiological processes to be fully felt at a pace the nervous system can metabolize.

How it can support you

Somatic Experiencing® allows survivors of pregnancy and infant loss to gently explore the imprints of loss in their body without becoming flooded by feelings, sensations, and other responses. Carrying our baby and then experiencing the loss of our baby is a complex, visceral experience. To know our body as the home where our baby once grew, and for some where our baby also died, may forever alter our relationship with it. However, with access to a body-inclusive practice like SE, over time, we may sense that our body is not solely a vessel of grief. For each of us, other unique layers coexist with the grief—layers that, once recognized, can serve as a counterbalance to our most tender pain. Those elements of our experience may not surface while we are in the deepest caverns of grief and often require spaciousness, patience, and rest to begin to emerge.

Importantly, SE does not rely on language alone. This is vital for loss that transcends words and is more fully expressed in sensations, emotions, and imagery. Over time, SE supports us in building a nuanced and intimate relationship with our bodies that not only allows us to process grief and loss but also reveals to us the deepest reservoirs within ourselves where strength, peace, and joy live. As we experience a greater embodied capacity to hold the full range of human experience, including our womb loss, without being undone by it, we can feel how our resilience naturally meets and grows around our wounds.

Centering Our Resilience After Womb Loss

A self-tending practice

In the wake of pregnancy and infant loss, many of us could write a long list of what our body knows about grief, loss, and/or trauma. While we can detail the nuances of the most painful experiences, moments, and realizations our body has archived, it is essential to remember that our bodies know as much about healing as they do about loss. They know as much about love as they do about grief. In fact, our bodies don't separate these qualities: healing lives alongside loss as much as love lives alongside grief. Nurturing the resilience that lives, breathes, and continuously emerges beneath and in response to our loss can thread together the parts of us that feel fragmented. So we can feel more integrated. So we can feel more whole.

In honor of your body's tremendous capacity to hold the full range of human experience and in alignment with the practice of SE, which centers resilience in how the body renegotiates trauma, I invite you to consider this question:

What does my body know about healing?

Your body may respond with silence. It may want to remind you of what it knows about loss and grief. With great compassion for yourself, pause to listen, notice, and honor what your body shares or does not share in this moment. After you've given your body some time and space to be present with its immediate experience, you might invite the question again:

What does my body know about healing?

Simply by asking it, this question plants a seed. Your body's healing insights may come to you later and at unexpected moments. Tending to this question with curiosity and trusting that your body *does* know about healing and how *you* heal is a beautiful way to reclaim your body as an ally, a confidant, and a *home* worthy of care, sweetness, and gentleness. It is empowering for your body, which may have been the central place you felt your loss, to also become the center of the wisdom that will accompany, bolster, and nourish you in your unique, nonlinear healing journey.

A Gentle Closing

Thank you for being here. For showing up for yourself, your body, and your grief as we explored this second threshold moment of birthing your loss. It is a moment worthy of careful consideration and deep sensitivity, even if we do not see this reflected in the world around us (yet). May you be gentle with yourself if you are making preparations to cross this threshold. Know that birth is a deeply embodied process, and it can be helpful to listen to what your body is calling for in any given moment. Your body wants what's best for you, even if this may be hard to hear right now. If you are reflecting back to this moment of birth, may you, too, be gentle with yourself as any thoughts, memories, or sensations arise.

As this chapter comes to a close, I invite you to pause for a few breaths with the closing verse to help you transition gently back into your life or to the next part of the book. And if anything in this chapter activated a strong response, consider doing something more to feel grounded. This may be an act of self-tending or reaching out to someone you trust for support. Honor what you need in this moment.

I am here, as I am.
And so it is.

You are here.
And we are with you.

CHAPTER 3

Enduring Your Loss

It's okay to rest.

The golden afternoon sunlight filtered in through a crack in the bathroom door, offering itself as a gentle companion to the soothing darkness that cocooned me. I had just given birth to my first pregnancy loss and was back in the shower, my baby's tiny body resting in a glass jar on the bathroom counter. I hadn't known to catch the remains, but I intuitively grabbed a sizable amount of tissue before it went down the drain. Upon further inspection, I could clearly make out features, such as tiny limbs and even a mouth with what looked like a tongue peeping out. I paused in awe of what I cradled in my hand. Following my body's lead, I returned to the shower in a daze. All I knew in that moment was how much I wanted to feel the cleansing warmth of a hot shower. At some point, my hand reached for the sugar scrub made by a friend, and I found myself gently and slowly rubbing it along my arms. My shoulders. My neck. My chest. And then over my belly, where I stayed a while. It was like a prayer, my hand reverently drawing circles over my womb—the subtle, sweet scent of vanilla flowing into my awareness and soothing me as I realized I was no longer pregnant. Knowing my friend's bright, beautiful energy was infused into the sugar scrub was comforting, helping me feel connected to her and less alone as I tended to this sensitive place.

~

In this chapter, we will consider common postpartum needs we face immediately after giving birth, after we've crossed the threshold from pregnant to no longer pregnant, and as our grief begins to blend with our postpartum time.

You, Too, Are Postpartum

The word *postpartum* simply means "after giving birth." This means anyone who has been pregnant and given birth is postpartum, including those of us who experience pregnancy and infant loss.[1] When I point out this important fact to those who have experienced womb loss, there is usually a pause as they realize the truth in it. It is not common for us to see ourselves as postpartum, nor is it something society recognizes. And once you are postpartum, you are always so. While the intensity of the acute postpartum time may fade, you and your body will continue to be in a postbirth state. It can never fully return to what was. We are in fact forever changed.

The following practice is an invitation to turn to your breath for support. It is an invitation to simplify the moment in the face of any overwhelm. It does this by inviting your attention to focus on two words and letting your body do what it knows how to already without conscious effort—breathe.

GROUNDING BREATHING PRACTICE

In-Out Breathing

The time after birthing our loss, especially immediately after, can so often be a period of overwhelming thoughts, feelings, and felt sensations. It can be a time of numbness, a sleepwalking kind of existence as you hold the dissonance between what you had expected/wanted/hoped and the reality of no longer being pregnant and having no child to bring home. May this breathing practice help you to feel grounded and more able to tend to your grieving and healing process.

The Invitation

From a comfortable position seated or lying down, start simply by noticing your breath. Noticing without any need to change it. You might notice where it enters your body—through your nose or through your mouth—and the subtle physical sensations as it does. You might notice how your body responds as your breath flows further into and then out of your body, as well as the parts of your body that move with it. You might also notice the rhythm of your breath. Is it fast, slow, or somewhere in between?

However your breath is right now, allow it to be as it is, without judgment or pressure to change it. Allow your inhalation and exhalation to last only as long as you want them to. Then, as you are ready, I invite you to think of the word *in* as you inhale and the word *out* as you exhale.

In

Out

In

Out

In

Out

These two simple words can be helpful, powerful anchors—something for your mind to hold on to when any given moment feels hard to endure. Continue to breathe with these words for as long as it feels right for you. When you are ready to bring this practice to a close, you can deepen your breath or press down with the parts of you touching the earth to help you transition.

Memory Making

As you consider the immediate time after giving birth, also consider what if any acts of memory making you would like to do with your baby, whether they died in the womb, during labor or birth, or while your baby is still alive. This can include looking at and holding them as well as bathing and dressing them. This can include capturing your brief time with them through photos or a video and creating lasting, tangible keepsakes to look back at later such as a photo book that can be shared with loved ones. There are even organizations like Now I Lay Me Down to Sleep that offer complimentary professional remembrance photography. If you are partnered, memory making can include them, and if you have living children, this can include them as well. If you are birthing in a hospital, you can inquire about options they have available, such as creating hand and foot molds or memory boxes. Memory making is about spending your time with the remains of your pregnancy, with the remains of your baby, in a way that is meaningful to you. It is also about capturing those moments in tangible ways to help you feel connected to those memories as time passes.

The following practice is an invitation to gain clarity about what acts of memory making may resonate with you. If you have already given birth, this practice may help you understand what you may have wanted at the time. This realization, even many years later, can help you tend to your grief now.

GROUNDING MINDFULNESS PRACTICE

A Tangible Connection

What we need in a given moment may not be clear to us until time has passed and we've had a chance to reflect. As frustrating as this may be when we want so much to have answers *now*, it can help to give ourselves time to gain the clarity we need. If you are preparing to birth, may the following support you in making meaningful decisions with what little time you will have with the remains of your pregnancy, with your baby. If you have already given birth, may the following support you in grieving what you may have wanted to help you remember your loss, your baby, and offer clarity for how you might memorialize your loss even now.

The Invitation

At your own pace, find your way into a comfortable resting position, either seated or lying down. Perhaps drape a blanket over your body to help yourself feel held in a warm embrace. Bring your awareness to your breath, gently following each inhalation and each exhalation, as your eyes soften or close. When you are ready, begin to imagine you are many years out from the birth of your loss—decades even. You might imagine what you look like, where you are, who you are with. This may be your lived reality now. Then, from that point in time, return to the memory of birthing your loss, your baby, and immediately after. Now, look down and imagine something appears in your hands, some tangible connection to that memory. Allow this item to emerge naturally, from the depths of your being. What do you see? Maybe it's a photo or a piece of clothing. Maybe it's jewelry with ashes cocooned inside. Stay here for a few more breaths, really taking in what is in your hands with your senses. Looking at it, touching it, maybe smelling it, or hugging it to your heart. When you are ready to bring this practice to a close, invite your breath to deepen to return you to the present moment, as you slowly open your eyes if they are closed.

Common Postpartum Changes

After giving birth vaginally or via a procedure, we are in transition yet again as our bodies work hard to return to a nonpregnant state while also grieving our womb loss. We are postpartum, and the following list of common postpartum experiences can apply to us too. These changes can feel like losses that need to be grieved. Loss of how your body was during pregnancy. Loss of how your body was before pregnancy. Please consult your health-care provider for guidance regarding care for your unique circumstances.

Tender perineum: After vaginal birth, your perineum (the skin between your vaginal opening and anus) can feel tender due to stretching or tearing in labor and stitches if they were needed. In lieu of wiping, you can use an angled peri bottle (a portable bidet) to ease any burning sensation while peeing and to gently clean without irritating the skin after using the toilet. Peri bottles help cleanse the perineum after all types of births in the days and weeks when your body releases the normal postbirth discharge known as lochia. Simply fill the bottle with warm water, sit on the toilet, squeeze the bottle, and direct the flow of water to your perineum while you urinate or have bowel movements and afterward to clean, then pat gently to dry or simply air dry. Witch hazel is known to offer cooling relief and can be added to the peri bottle. Other comfort measures include applying ice packs or instant cooling maxi pads, witch hazel pad liners, sprays or foam, and soaking in a sitz bath with Epsom salt for a few minutes to help relieve discomfort.

Postpartum contractions: Also known as afterpains, afterbirth pains, or postpartum cramping, postpartum contractions can be felt for several days after all types of birth as the uterus contracts to return to its nonpregnant size and state. The contracting and relaxing of your uterine muscles also protects you from losing too much blood (i.e., postpartum hemorrhage) from the wound where the placenta was once attached to the uterine wall.[2] If you were pregnant long enough for your body to produce milk, lactating can signal the release of the hormone oxytocin, which can increase cramping. Such cramps can feel intense for some and very painful for others. To help ease the pain of postpartum contractions, you can ask your health-care provider about pain-relief medication, take a walk, apply a heated pad to your belly, or turn to the same comfort measures used to cope with contractions during labor, such as breathing or relaxation practices.

Postpartum vaginal bleeding: Postpartum contractions also help the uterus release lochia to return to a nonpregnant state and prepare for menstruation in a process called uterine involution. Uterine involution begins immediately after all births and can last for four to six weeks or longer. More than blood, lochia includes mucus, uterine and placental tissue, and bacteria. The discharge is usually heavy to start, then eases over time, with the color lightening from dark red to pink or brown and then white or yellow with a mucus texture.[3] Consider using more absorbent maxi pads to accommodate the heavy flow that can accompany pregnancy and infant loss (avoid inserting anything into the vagina to prevent infection, usually until six weeks after birth or until your health-care provider confirms it's safe), and consider postpartum mesh underwear for comfort and breathability.

Pain after cesarean birth: It is common to feel fatigue and incision soreness. Just as with any birth and just as with any major surgery, rest is essential. You can ask your health-care provider for pain-relief medication and your loved ones for support so you can rest. Take care to hydrate to replace fluids in the body as C-sections also include blood loss.

Postpartum hemorrhoids: After pregnancy, changes in blood flow and the added pressure from pushing during a vaginal birth can cause the veins in and around your lower rectum and anus to become irritated and swollen. Witch hazel is a common go-to for easing the discomfort of hemorrhoids. Consider applying witch hazel pads or foam or topical steroid creams; soaking in a sitz bath; and increasing your fiber intake to prevent constipation.

Breast tenderness, soreness, and leaking: Depending on how long you carried your pregnancy, your body may produce milk, and giving birth can signal to your body that it is time to share it. In the context of womb loss, this may feel shocking, uncomfortable, and unfair if you had wanted a healthy, living infant to feed. Consider using nursing pads to absorb leaking milk. Later in the chapter, we will explore lactation after loss more.

Shifts in mood: It is normal not to feel like yourself in the postpartum time, due in part to the sudden decrease in the hormones estrogen and progesterone as well as factors like a lack of sleep, nutritious food, and support. Commonly referred to as "baby blues," mood changes immediately postpartum can include feeling tired, depressed, anxious, sad, irritable, unable to focus, unable to sleep, and a desire to cry for seemingly no reason. Such feeling states are considered normal within the first two to three weeks after birthing living children; external support is recommended if they last beyond that time. In womb loss, however, these same changes reflect natural grief responses and can last well beyond two weeks. It is difficult, if impossible, to distinguish between what is strictly a natural postpartum response and what is a natural grief response, as both are intertwined.

Perinatal Mood and Anxiety Disorders (PMADs): PMADs is an umbrella term to describe mental health conditions that are more severe and shifts in mood that are longer lasting during and up to a year after pregnancy, conditions that make it difficult to function in daily life or even to continue living. In the United States alone, an estimated one in seven pregnant and postpartum women are affected by PMADs regardless of income, with depressive symptoms affecting 40 to 60 percent of low-income women.[4] If you suspect you are suffering from any of these conditions, please reach out to someone you trust like a health-care provider, a family member, a friend, or a confidential helpline like that run by Postpartum Support International. You absolutely do not need to manage any of these severe symptoms alone. There is support for you. Please see chapter 8 and the resources section for more information on PMADs.

Postpartum hair loss: This often comes as a surprise and yet is a common experience caused by hormone changes. The rise in the hormone estrogen during pregnancy keeps you from shedding as much hair as usual, and when estrogen levels drop after birth, it is as if your body is catching up to shed all the hair it didn't while you were pregnant.[5] While it is considered temporary, this may feel especially distressing as it is yet another loss and one that may make it harder feel comfortable in your body.

Stretch marks: These are actually scars that develop on areas like the abdomen, breasts, hips, and buttocks once your skin stretches to accommodate a pregnancy. They may feel itchy and may not go away, though they may fade. This can be another reminder of your womb loss and make it challenging to nurture a softer relationship with your body.

Constipation: Another common postpartum experience, even in womb loss, is infrequent and uncomfortable or even painful bowel movements due to factors such as hemorrhoids and shifts in hormones. To help your body have a bowel movement, you can consume foods and drinks that are high in fiber (e.g., prune juice), drink plenty of water, and rest. Over-the-counter stool softeners, laxatives, and enemas can help in more severe cases.

Diastasis recti: You may still look pregnant even after your body has physically released the pregnancy. This is normal and common, and while your body will naturally begin to shift back to a nonpregnant state, there is much that can be done to support your body in this process, including resting, sleeping, eating nutrient-rich food, moving gently, feeling emotionally supported, and receiving caring touch such as postpartum massage and postpartum abdominal wrapping. It is also common to develop diastasis recti, which is when the abdominal muscles separate after being stretched during pregnancy. This can cause the belly to continue to bulge months or even years after birth, which can be a difficult physical reminder of womb loss. You can heal diastasis recti with gentle, specialized exercises to help close the separation; a pelvic floor physical therapist can support you with this.

Postpartum healing and grieving are each intense processes on their own. To endure them simultaneously in womb loss demands much of us. As your body endures any of these common postpartum experiences in addition to carrying your grief, it can be hard to simply be in your body let alone try to understand what you are feeling. And yet, being able to identify what you are feeling is an essential part of healing. The following is a practice that invites you to connect to your body and name what you are feeling. Doing so can help you get the support you need.

GROUNDING REFLECTION PRACTICE

Feeling Words

Imagine being in a room with multiple *yous*. Each *you* embodies a distinct feeling. Naming what we feel is like inviting each *you* to come forward and be recognized, maybe even offering that *you* a warm embrace. As this part of you feels seen and reassured, it doesn't need to work so hard to get your attention and can feel safe softening. In this way, simply identifying what you feel has the power to heal.

The Invitation

Begin in any seated form that feels right for your body, perhaps pressing down into the parts of you that are touching a surface or the earth, feeling a sense of grounding as you do. Then I invite you to bring your awareness to your breath, perhaps taking a few deep breaths to help your mind release other thoughts. Remember you can return to your breath or actively press down into the earth to help you feel grounded at any point in this reflection practice, and beyond.

When it feels right, begin to read through the following list of words and circle or highlight those that resonate with you in this moment. You may feel an energetic tug toward certain words. You may tear up or begin to cry when you read others. You may read some and not feel any sort of reaction. I invite you to embody compassion for yourself as you name what you feel without judgment, letting your feelings be known without pressure to change them. There is no right or wrong way to feel, and it is natural to embody many different feelings at once, even conflicting ones. And your feelings may change, with some becoming stronger or less present. You might revisit this reflection practice in the coming days, weeks, or months and see how your internal landscape shifts with time.

And perhaps consider words in other languages that may better express your grief. Much like I felt a strong resonance with the words *nakunan* and *nakuanan,* you, too, may find that another language speaks more truthfully to the heart of your experience. You might also write down words that you feel but do not see listed.

Abandoned	Curious	Hateful	Miserable
Alone	Cynical	Heard	Numb
Angry	Depressed	Held	Okay
Anguished	Desperate	Helpful	Overwhelmed
Anxious	Disconnected	Helpless	Pained
Apathetic	Discouraged	Hopeless	Panicky
Appreciated	Demoralized	Hurt	Patient
Appreciative	Distrustful	Inadequate	Peaceful
Ashamed	Distracted	Incapable	Pessimistic
Awkward	Doubtful	Impatient	Playful
Betrayed	Embarrassed	Inferior	Powerful
Bitter	Empty	Insignificant	Powerless
Broken	Enraged	Insecure	Preoccupied
Calm	Excited	Intelligent	Proud
Capable	Exhausted	Isolated	Reassured
Centered	Fearful	Jealous	Reflective
Cherished	Foggy	Joyful	Regretful
Compassionate	Foolish	Judgmental	Rejected
Confident	Forgotten	Lethargic	Relieved
Conflicted	Frustrated	Lonely	Resentful
Confused	Grateful	Lost	Resigned
Content	Grounded	Loved	Resilient
Creative	Guilty	Loving	Resistant
Critical	Happy	Mad	Respected

Sad	Stressed	Traumatized	Wanted
Satisfied	Supported	Trusting	Weak
Scared	Surprised	Uninterested	Weird
Sentimental	Tearful	Unseen	Worthless
Sexy	Terrified	Unsure	Worthy
Shocked	Thankful	Upset	
Sleepy	Tired	Valued	

An Additional Invitation: Honoring Both/And

It is natural to embody multiple and even seemingly contradictory feelings at one time. Allow every feeling to be acknowledged. All are valid and honored here. If you circled or highlighted any conflicting feelings, take a moment to write them in the following format to help affirm them for yourself:

I feel _____ *and* _____.

Mint Cacao Tea

A Recipe by Nora Vitaliani

The following recipe is one offered with great tenderness as it pertains to the issue of lactating after loss—a topic that so often catches people by surprise and that will be addressed in greater detail in the next section. If your body is producing milk and you prefer that it not, this recipe is an offering to support you. It comes from a friend and gifted chef whose food and drinks have nourished me deeply while attending retreats for bereaved mothers offered by Return to Zero: HOPE. Nora helped me understand just how healing fresh, seasonal food can be for a grieving and postpartum body like mine. Truly, each time I ate her food or tasted her teas, I closed my eyes and felt the life energy of the ingredients tend to my body and renew my spirit. And I was reminded of what a tremendous relief it is to have someone tend to my dietary needs with care. I felt seen and held, and I hope this recipe can help you feel the same.

Peppermint has long been regarded as an herbal support for decreasing milk production as well as relieving painful menstrual cramps and fatigue, improving concentration, and helping relax the body. In this simple recipe, peppermint is combined with another ancient healing plant, cacao, which is revered for its ability to soften the heart and lift the mood. Nutrient- and antioxidant-rich honey is also included to support your body in healing after pregnancy and birth.

- 1 tablespoon dried peppermint leaves (or 3 tea bags)
- 1 tablespoon cacao powder
- 32 ounces boiling water
- Honey (or sweetener of choice)
- Milk of choice

Stir peppermint leaves and cacao powder into hot water and let steep for 15 minutes. Strain into a quart mason jar. Add honey and milk to taste. As you hold the drink in your hand and notice the scents floating up to meet you, perhaps take a moment to allow any tension in your face, neck, and shoulders to melt away. It may feel hard to be in your body, especially if it is producing milk for a child you want but cannot tend to. And while it may feel like your body is betraying you in this way, know that it is responding to a natural physical progression of the postbirth time. May the warmth of this drink and the healing force of its ingredients soften your connection to your body so that you may tend to it—to yourself—with the compassion both deserve. The tea can be served hot or cold and kept in the refrigerator for up to a week.

Alternative tea to support lactation suppression

- 1 tablespoon dried peppermint leaves or a handful of fresh mint leaves
- 1 sprig fresh rosemary
- 32 ounces boiling water

Put the herbs into hot water and steep for up to 15 minutes. Strain and serve hot or cold.

Including Living Children

If you have living children, it can be meaningful to invite them to join you in the hospital room or at home to see or even touch their sibling. Having this tangible experience with your womb loss can offer an opportunity for them to feel connected, ask questions, process their grief, and better understand your grief. In completing the Holding Space for Pregnancy Loss training with Amy Wright Glenn—chaplain, womb loss survivor, and founder of the Institute for the Study of Birth, Breath, and Death—I heard a story and saw precious photos that left a deep impression. I share it here with Amy's permission. A mother had given birth to her stillborn child in a hospital and wanted her living daughters to meet their sibling. In a simple yet powerful ritual that they intuitively created, they decided to paint all the children's fingers with the same color nail polish. Seeing photos of this moment—one of the baby's painted toes and one of the living children standing and looking down at the baby—moved me so deeply it took my breath away. As you consider how to spend the short time you have with your baby, invite your living children to join you and create memories together. If your living children express uncertainty, you might ask the hospital staff for support. If they feel strongly about not seeing the baby, it is important to honor that too.

It's also important to use language with living children, especially younger ones, that is clear and tangible in lieu of euphemisms that may leave them wondering or confused. For example, you might say, "Our baby died inside my body because their body didn't have what it needed to continue growing," instead of saying, "The baby is sleeping." The latter may lead to younger living children feeling scared to sleep for fear of not waking up or scared for their loved ones to sleep for the same reason. It can also help to reassure younger living children if they express fear about dying or people they love dying. You might say, "Yes, it is sad and scary to know that we will all die, *and* there are things we can do to keep our bodies safe and healthy so we can live longer, like wear our seatbelts and eat food that helps our bodies." You can also ask staff for support in how to talk to your living children about the loss and what they can do to create memories with their sibling. It can also be helpful to read children's books about pregnancy and infant loss; you will find some recommendations in the resources section at the back of this book.

The following practice invites you to offer yourself the warmth and gentle touch you are worthy of receiving. And it is one that you can teach to even the youngest of living children, helping them to build their own toolbox of grounding practices that they can turn to in difficult moments.

GROUNDING EMBODIMENT PRACTICE

Warming Hands

This seemingly simple embodiment practice can be a powerful self-tending tool to add to your toolbox for moments when you want to feel more grounded. More centered. More at ease. Although your body is intimately connected to your loss, know that your body can also be a tool for healing and a place of healing.

The Invitation

When you are ready, find your way into a comfortable seated position. Perhaps take a moment to press down into your sit bones and feet to actively ground yourself. Invite your awareness to follow your breath flowing in and out of your body, releasing any other thoughts for now. In your own time, bring the palms of your hands to touch and rub them together to create warmth. Then gently rest the palms of your hands over your eyes, allowing your eyes to close if that feels right for you. And breathe, feeling the warmth you created for yourself. With your hands over your eyes, you might explore a gentle rocking of your body, forward and backward or side to side. When you are ready to bring this practice to a close, you can lower your hands to your lap, slowly open your eyes if they are closed, and take a deep cleansing breath or press into the earth.

Lactation After Loss

Another aspect of womb loss that is often shocking is the fact that your milk might come in, depending on how far along your pregnancy progressed.

As mentioned earlier, lactation after loss can feel unfair. You have milk to give, but your baby is not alive to drink it. Or in the case of infant loss when your baby is alive for some time in the neonatal intensive care unit (NICU), you may find yourself trying to increase your milk production and expressing often to feed your baby before they die. There are a few options you can consider if you are lactating after loss:

- You can choose to express (pump) milk to donate (also known as *bereavement pumping*) to a milk bank or to other families in your community to help provide optimal nutrition for infants who don't have access to breast milk, including premature and sick infants in hospitals. Some womb loss survivors may find this helps with their grief as a meaningful way to honor their loss, their baby, as well as helping others. But if milk donation does not resonate with you, that is completely okay.

- You can choose to decrease your milk production until it stops completely (also known as *lactation suppression*). This includes expressing just enough milk to lessen engorgement (which can be painful) applying cold compresses, and taking over-the-counter medication for any pain. Nursing pads can be used to absorb any leaking milk. You may find it helpful to connect with a lactation consultant who can offer you personalized support, particularly one who specializes in supporting those who have experienced pregnancy and infant loss. You can find more information online via organizations like La Leche League International.

- You can choose to try expressing before suppressing, allowing yourself a chance to see how it feels to actually express milk before deciding whether to continue and donate or suppress. You may express milk for a living infant, and after they die, choose to donate what remains or hold on to it if that feels right to you. Consider, too, that you can express milk to keep for your own memory making, such as using it for breast milk keepsake jewelry (where your breast milk is protected in the jewelry itself) or for mourning rituals like a milk bath (see below).

The following practice is a special offering from my friend Nicole Longmire, a bereaved mother and International Board Certified Lactation Consultant. It can support you in grieving your womb loss and the loss of your breastfeeding experience if that is one you had wanted.

GROUNDING RITUAL PRACTICE

Milk Ceremony for Womb Loss

This simple ceremony is a way to say goodbye to and grieve the loss of your lactation journey.

You will need the following:

- Expressed milk if your milk has come in or alternative milk
- A cup to hold the milk
- A large bowl (this can be a special one that has meaning for you)
- Soft lighting if indoors (e.g., candles), calming music, essential oils

The Invitation

This special milk ceremony is an invitation to reconnect with your baby and the precious milk that was meant to nourish them. This can be done alone, with your partner, your living children, or with another trusted person like a doula. There is no right or wrong way to do this. You may follow the suggestions below or use your intuition to make this ceremony your own.

1. Find a quiet place indoors or outdoors to do the ceremony. If indoors, you are welcome to create a soothing environment by using soft lighting, calming music, and even the power of essential oils whether with a diffuser or by placing a few drops onto a napkin.

2. Place the milk in a cup or special container.

3. With your hands hovering over the large bowl, slowly pour the milk over your hands or have another person do this for you. Wash your hands in this sacred milk, noticing how it feels on your skin, as you

gently rub your hands together and allow thoughts, feelings, and memories to naturally emerge. If you are doing this outdoors, you can allow the milk you pour over your hands to fall directly onto the earth. Perhaps into a special memory garden, at the site where your baby is buried, or another meaningful location. Consider taking photos or a video to memorialize this moment.

Words of Comfort

Even the simplest, shortest expressions of condolences have the power to heal and soften the pain of our loss. Unfortunately, in a grief-avoidant society like ours, we lack strong cultural guidelines for how to support those who survive womb loss, and many if not most people do not yet know to offer us their condolences. We see this reality reflected in the greeting cards available for sale. Greeting cards reveal a lot about what a culture values. They are a way to say *this is worth acknowledging*. I am often in the greeting card section of stores looking for those that speak to womb loss. Not surprisingly, they are hard to come by, and the cards in the pregnancy, more often labeled "baby," section focus on babies expected to be born alive and thrive. The fact that it is hard to find greeting cards that celebrate and honor the one carrying the pregnancy reflects the lack of attention given to the postpartum period as well—to the healing those who carry pregnancies must go through after the hard labor of gestating, laboring, and birthing. But this can change. And it can start with us.

Having your loss acknowledged with even the simplest phrase can be incredibly healing. And having it acknowledged in a way that feels comforting to you can be even better. The following practice is an invitation to identify phrases that resonate with you so that your support network may know how to offer condolences and words of comfort that are sensitive to you and your grief.

Comforting Phrases

People around us, even those who care deeply for us, may not know what to say or do when they learn we have experienced such a loss. They may feel uncomfortable. They may feel their own grief rising up within them. Or they may say or do things that we experience as hurtful or insensitive despite their best intentions. May the following support you in tending to your emotional needs and, in turn, tending to our collective needs.

The Invitation

When you are ready, read through the following list of phrases and circle or highlight those that would feel comforting to hear someone say to you. Alternatively, you might ask a partner or other support person to read each phrase to you so you can see in real time how it feels to hear it.

- I'm sorry.
- I'm sorry for your loss.
- I'm very sorry that your baby died.
- I'm sorry that [baby's name] died.
- I offer my deepest condolences for your loss.
- I'm sorry for all you've been through and are going through still.
- I'm here for you.
- I'm thinking of you and sending my love.
- I'm not sure what to do, but I'm here for you.
- It's okay to cry.
- It's okay to grieve.
- It's not your fault.
- I can't take away your pain, but I'll be with you while you feel it.
- You don't have to be okay.
- How are you feeling today?

- Whatever you feel is okay.
- What you're going through is so hard.
- I see you doing the best you can.
- You are not alone.
- You can cry for as long as you need.
- May I give you a hug?
- May I sit with you?
- Would you like to talk?
- Would you like to hold my hand?
- Would you like to go for a walk?

You are welcome to add any phrases that resonate for you but aren't listed here. How did it feel to read through those phrases or to hear them read aloud to you? How did your body respond?

After you have finished, you might consider sharing this with someone you trust who can then share this information with others in your life if you choose to share the news of your loss. This may look like writing your preferred phrases on a piece of paper and taping it to the hospital door or the front door of your home. Or you might write them on index cards and ask guests to read through the cards before coming in to see you. Please keep in mind that what feels supportive to you now may not later as your needs and preferences shift. You might make note of other phrases you come across and add them to your list of comforting phrases.

Offering from the Collective

The following is an offering from one of the sweetest spirits I know. Princess and I met several years ago when she wrapped my belly in the Malaysian tradition of Bengkung after my fourth pregnancy. Her kind presence, warm smile, and words of affirmation helped me feel at ease despite all the discomfort and exhaustion I felt in my postbirth body and the grief I continued to carry from my two womb losses. To see and feel someone take the time to wrap you lovingly in this way is a gift. There's a palpable reverence with each pass of the cloth, and it's hard not to feel like you are being recognized in that moment for all you have been through. Months later, Princess and her team of BelliBind doulas were present at one of my Our Womb Loss dining events, offering guests their very own private belly-wrapping session in honor of them and their postpartum bodies. To mourn them and their womb losses. Because, like you, they deserved heartfelt condolences and gentle touch sensitive to their needs as postpartum and bereaved.

AN OFFERING BY PRINCESS ESTOCIA MCKINNEY

Bengkung Belly Binding

What it is

Bengkung belly binding is a traditional postpartum practice from Malaysia, though cultures around the globe, from Haiti to Japan and even colonial America, practice some form of abdominal binding after birth (also known as belly wrapping). Belly-wrapping practices are rooted in ancient wisdom, passed down through generations, and symbolize a return to yourself after the profound experience of carrying a pregnancy. In the sacred tradition of Bengkung belly binding, the Bengkung—a long strip of cloth—is gently and lovingly wrapped around the postpartum belly, starting from the hips and moving upward, knotting it carefully each time the cloth returns to center. With each graceful movement of the fabric, the womb space is enveloped in a cocoon of warmth and support reminiscent of a protective and loving embrace. The gentle hug that belly wrapping provides can support your uterus as it shrinks to its pre-pregnancy size, assist the mending of abdominal muscles that have separated during pregnancy to accommodate a growing belly, help your organs as they return to their original positions, and encourage safe posture by supporting the back and pelvic floor. This long-standing postpartum tradition also nurtures a spiritual connection by encouraging the wearer to reconnect with their body, listen to its whispers, and honor its needs.

How it can support you

The traditional art of Bengkung binding can be a loving form of physical, emotional, and spiritual support for those who have experienced pregnancy and infant loss, even months or years later. Its benefits can include the following:

Physical Comfort: Pregnancy loss can leave physical changes and discomfort. Bengkung belly binding offers gentle compression to aid in postpartum physical recovery and provides a comforting feeling of being held during this challenging time.

Symbolic Significance: Wrapping the belly can symbolize connection to the pregnancy that ended or to the baby that died and also a sense of closure. It acknowledges the existence of the baby and the experience of motherhood, even in the absence of a living child.

Emotional Healing: Bengkung belly binding can foster self-love amidst the emotional devastation that pregnancy and infant loss can bring, allowing individuals to focus on themselves with tenderness and in a meditative process. Ritualizing the recovery from womb loss is a beautiful way to honor your body and yourself.

Spiritual Connection: Many cultures view belly binding as a spiritual practice. It honors the sacred vessel that carried the child's soul and helps connect the individual with personal, cultural, or spiritual beliefs. Prayers, affirmations, or mindfulness rituals accompany the binding, adding deeper meaning.

Community: Trained birth workers like midwives and belly-binding specialists can offer gentle connection and recovery guidance as they wrap your postbirth body. Loved ones can also complete training to learn how to do belly binding safely. This sense of togetherness can provide great comfort.

Empowerment: Pregnancy and infant loss so often lead to a feeling of powerlessness. Bengkung belly binding can restore a sense of autonomy as you choose to have someone wrap your belly or as you dedicate time and energy to learn how to properly self-wrap and tend to your womb space.

Continued Self-Tending: The practice extends beyond immediate recovery and can become a regular self-tending ritual nurturing physical, emotional, and spiritual healing over time. Each pass of the cloth is an invitation to remember the strength and resilience that exists within you, transforming the act into a meditation of self-love.

A Gentle Womb-Love Meditation Practice

A self-tending practice

As a restorative offering, womb-love meditations can be powerful tools to help navigate this challenging time with gentleness for yourself and all you have been through. The following is a womb-love meditation to support your grieving and healing process. Follow what resonates and know that you can adjust it to fit your needs.

1. Find a Quiet and Comfortable Space: Choose a peaceful and quiet place where you won't be disturbed. You can sit or lie down, whichever is more comfortable for you.

2. Set Your Intention: Begin by setting your intention for the meditation. You might say something like, "I am here to honor my womb and the loss I've experienced. I invite love and healing energy into my body."

3. Take Deep Breaths: Close your eyes and take several deep, slow breaths. Inhale deeply through your nose, allowing your abdomen to rise, and exhale slowly through your mouth, releasing any tension with each breath.

4. Connect with Your Womb: If it feels okay, gently place your hands on your lower abdomen, where your womb is located. If you feel uncomfortable bringing touch to this area, you can hover your hands in front of it instead or place them over your heart. Feel the warmth or energy of your hands connecting with this sacred space.

5. Visualize Healing Light: Imagine a soft, warm, healing light radiating from your hands into your womb. Picture this light as a soothing and loving energy that's there to heal and nurture you.

6. Send Love: Connect to your womb with kindness using thoughts or words said aloud. You can say something as simple as, "I am here for you," "Thank you for the life you carried," or "I honor the journey we are on together."

7. Release: As you continue to breathe deeply, visualize any emotions or energy you want to release leaving your body with each exhalation. Give yourself permission to release or to simply soften any guilt, pain, or sadness you may be holding on to.

8. Nurture and Rebuild: Imagine your womb being gently cradled and nurtured by the healing light. See it becoming strong, healthy, and filled with love.

9. Repeat an Affirmation: Repeat an affirmation that resonates with you, for example:

    "I am worthy of love and healing."

    "I am learning to trust my body's wisdom and its ability to heal."

    "I am surrounded by love and support."

10. Stay in the Moment: Spend some time in this meditative state, allowing yourself to feel whatever emotions arise without judgment. Be gentle with yourself.

11. Closing: When you are ready to bring the meditation to a close, slowly bring your awareness back to your surroundings. Wiggle your fingers and toes, and open your eyes.

12. Self-Tending: After the meditation, engage in activities that nourish your body and spirit. This could include taking a warm bath, journaling your thoughts and feelings, spending time in nature, lighting a candle, placing a heating pad over your belly, or wrapping this sacred part of you.

Remember that healing takes time, and it's okay to seek additional support from a therapist, pregnancy-and-infant-loss coach, support group, or other trusted person. Be patient with yourself, and know you are resilient and have the capacity to tend to your body and spirit on this healing journey.

A Gentle Closing

Thank you for being here. For showing up for yourself, your body, and your grief as we explored this third threshold moment of transitioning from being pregnant to no longer being pregnant and the acute postpartum time. It is a tremendous yet often unacknowledged moment when your grief begins to intersect with your postpartum needs. May you be gentle with yourself as you process what this moment means and feels like to you. And know that it's okay to rest. You have been through so much already.

As this chapter comes to a close, I invite you to pause for a few breaths and with the closing verse to help you transition gently back into your life or to the next part of the book. And if anything in this chapter activated a strong response, consider doing something more to feel grounded. This may be an act of self-tending or reaching out to someone you trust for support. Honor what you need in this moment.

I am here, as I am.
And so it is.

You are here.
And we are with you.

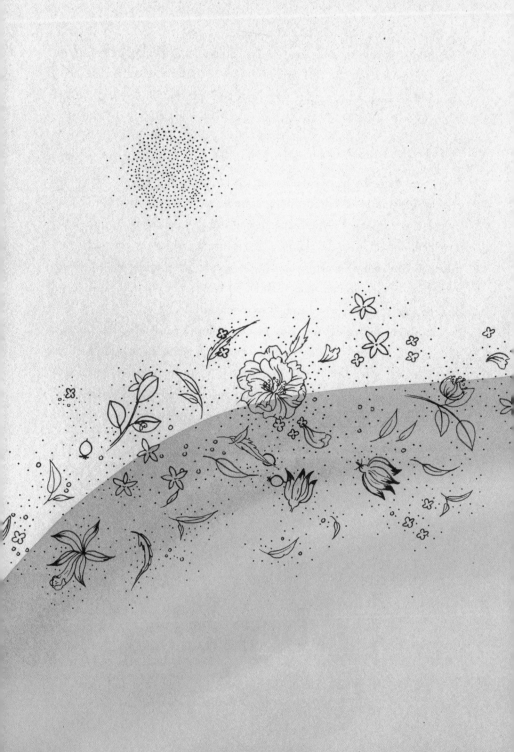

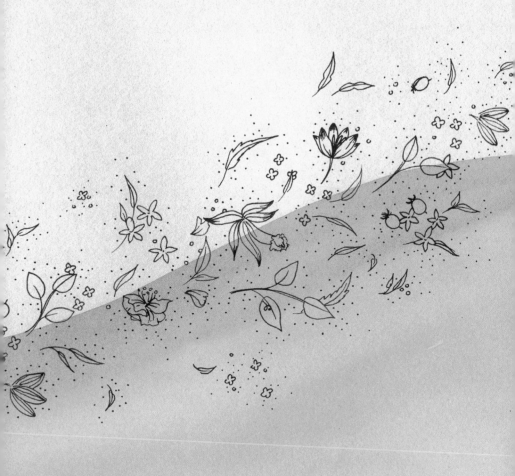

part two

our grief

CHAPTER 4

Grief in the Postpartum Time

Where does it hurt?

I first met Jessica in 2016. I had recently moved back home to Southern California after spending the majority of my twenties living in Chicago, and I was eager to connect with other marriage and family therapists. I still remember how Jessica's kind smile welcomed me and how inviting her office felt that afternoon as the soft, golden sunlight flowed in through the windows.

Though it was our first time meeting, there was a shared feeling of warmth, and in the course of our conversation, I learned that Jessica had recently experienced a miscarriage. She described how her sister, who was living on the East Coast, had sent her a care package that included a shawl. The air was thick with emotion as Jessica described how, when she put the shawl around her shoulders, it felt like a big, warm hug from her sister.

It was as if time stopped for that moment as I felt the vibration of her emotions in her words and saw the weight of them in her eyes. I could imagine the sensation of wrapping a shawl around my own shoulders and the comfort it would offer. The permission it would give me to cry. And in that moment with Jessica, the tears in my eyes mirrored her own.

~

It would be months before I learned firsthand what womb loss could entail. How it and the ensuing grief would feel in my body. I had no personal connection to the topic, no point of reference for the pain she was sharing.

And still, her story and how meaningful the shawl was to her moved me. Even now, many years later, I find myself tearing up as I think back to that moment and the shawl that was such a simple but powerful gift.

Oftentimes, it is the simplest acts done with great love that are the most comforting and leave the deepest impressions. The power is in the acknowledgment and validation the gift offers and how it can help give us permission to grieve.

Grieving Is Feeling

Grief is what you feel in response to a loss, whether it is a death or a non-death loss (like the ending of a relationship or the loss of an ability). Simply put, grieving is feeling, allowing yourself to feel what a loss means to you. The greater the meaning, the deeper the feelings. The deeper the feelings, the more the loss influences your life. While it is common to think of grief as something negative that we need to get rid of, get over, or get past, we can instead think of grief more neutrally this way, and we can also consider the wide spectrum of feelings that our grief can encompass. Grief can feel like love as much as it can feel like pain, for at its essence, grief is connection. In womb loss, grief is connection to our pregnancy that ended. Connection to our baby who died. Connection to our bodies that have endured so much to transition from being not pregnant to pregnant and back again. If coping with womb loss feels hard, that is completely understandable. You were pregnant, you labored, you gave birth, and now you are postpartum while you are grieving. You are recovering from a series of intense full-being experiences while also feeling what your womb loss means to you. That is a lot.

Grieving is feeling, and feeling can be hard. Sometimes it is so hard that we may pull away, distract, or numb to protect ourselves from being overwhelmed, to help us survive. Yet what we feel in response to a loss that is meaningful remains within us until we are ready to feel it fully and acknowledge the part of us that is carrying it. The following practice invites you to use your breath to tend to your grief. To help your grief soften rather than harden. To help the part of you that is grieving feel witnessed rather than alone.

Letting Your Breath Meet Your Grief

As with all the practices shared here, remember that you are in full control. If you notice any discomfort beginning to manifest in your body, consider doing something to feel grounded before continuing. This can include deepening your breath or physically pressing down into the ground. If grounding practices do not seem to help, it may be your body's way of asking you to take a break. It's okay to listen to your body's cues and honor your needs. In fact, it is supported and encouraged.

The Invitation

When you are ready, find a comfortable position seated or lying down and consider draping a blanket over your body to help you feel warm and safely held—perhaps tucking the sides of the blanket under your body for a felt sense of being cocooned. Taking your time, bring your attention to your breath, allowing your body to breathe naturally, without effort. Then begin to notice where your grief is stored in your body. These might be places that are holding tension or areas that are aching. Pause in each place and allow your breath to meet your grief, to be with it like a kind friend, ready to hold this part of you with care. If it helps, you can imagine your inhalation tinted in a color that feels soothing and allow that color to flow in to your grief. Let it surround your grief in a gentle embrace. If it feels accessible to you, continue to breathe into this part of your body until you feel a noticeable softening. Perhaps allow your breath to match the depth of your grief—the deeper the grief, the deeper the breath. Acknowledgment is powerful medicine and can soften even the most hardened parts of us. Let your breath offer gentle acknowledgment to the grief within you. When you are ready to bring this practice to a close, you can take a deep, cleansing breath and wiggle your toes and fingers to help return you to the present moment.

Grieving Your Way

There is no right or wrong way to grieve. Remember, grieving is feeling, and what you feel in response to your womb loss is unique to you. Common grief responses include but are not limited to the following, which is adapted from a list by Our House Grief Support Center to more specifically reflect womb loss and the nuances of pregnancy and the postpartum period.[1]

Grief can be experienced emotionally

- Sadness or deep sorrow, including sadness for the end of the fertility journey
- A sense of helplessness, including a sense of powerlessness regarding fertility
- A sense of hopelessness and even feeling life may not be worth living
- Fear that you or someone else you know will die or that future pregnancies may end in loss
- Anger that the pregnancy ended in loss or the death of your baby; anger at your baby for leaving you; anger at health-care providers or the health-care systems that you turned to for support; anger about insensitive comments made by others
- Guilt about something you did or did not do, often under the premise that the pregnancy or infant loss could have been prevented
- Longing for one more moment with your baby or to return to the time before womb loss was confirmed
- Major mood changes (see chapter 8 for more on perinatal mood and anxiety disorders)

Grief can be experienced physically or behaviorally

- Changes in eating or sleeping
- Difficulty functioning on a daily basis
- Emptiness or pain felt in the body (pain can also be attributed to physical exertion during pregnancy, birth, and the postpartum period)

- Difficulty being still
- Feeling exhausted or a lack of energy (can also be connected to fluctuating hormones during pregnancy and after birth)
- Crying that can occur unexpectedly and include sudden, powerful waves of emotion, also known as "grief bursts" (a common symptom of "baby blues")
- Distracted behaviors, including keeping busy, self-harm, or addiction
- Reminiscing about pregnancy/baby by telling stories or looking at pictures or other mementos

Grief can be experienced cognitively

- Hard to believe pregnancy has ended, the baby has died, that you have experienced womb loss
- Forgetfulness (research shows that a woman's brain may change more quickly and drastically during pregnancy and in the postpartum period than any other time in her life, causing forgetfulness and significant shifts in mood)[2]
- Difficulty concentrating
- Questioning why the pregnancy ended, why the baby died, and may be intensely focused on seeking answers
- Feeling stuck in a cycle of negative thoughts related to the womb loss (ruminating)

Grief can be experienced spiritually

- Searching for meaning and questioning your life's purpose
- Questioning or strengthening values or religious beliefs
- A sense of the baby's presence, including feeling phantom kicks and dreaming of the baby

Grief and grieving can easily and often be overwhelming—all-consuming even. It can help to tend to our grief with short but meaningful grounding practices. The following practice is an invitation to access your resilience and tend to your grief with a comforting memory.

Remembering a Moment of Comfort

The feelings that we have felt throughout our lifetime can be felt again through the practice and power of remembering. May the following allow your mind to connect to a comforting memory and infuse your body with that feeling once more. And may this offer you a gentle reprieve from the harder parts of your grief.

The Invitation

When you are ready, find your way into a comfortable resting position and perhaps soften your gaze or close your eyes. Allow any thoughts to melt away as you bring your awareness to your breath or to the sensation of your body touching the earth or other surface you're resting on. Then begin to recall a time when someone comforted you. You don't need to try too hard. Simply allow a memory to surface, and once one does, explore this memory with your senses. What do you see? What do you hear? What do you smell? What do you taste? What do you feel? You might recall how old you were, where you were, the time of day. Who were you with, and what did they do that helped you feel comforted? Can you recall with your body what you felt in that moment as you received their care? You are welcome to stay with this memory for as long as it feels right, and when this visualization practice feels complete, you can take a deep cleansing breath to help return you to the present moment.

It is said that love never dies. The loving care that someone shared with you in the memory you revisited for this practice is still very much alive and available to you. Whenever you feel alone in your grief, know that you can access the care that was shared with you in this memory or others like it.

And know that to choose to access the felt experience of such memories is a testament to your innate resilience and your capacity to tend to your needs. Enduring womb loss is hard. It is hard, *and* you have the resilience and tools to endure.

Your Loss Is Real and Your Grief Is Valid

Pregnancy and infant loss are not typically acknowledged with the same depth of condolence and reverence as other forms of loss or death. Instead, they are all too often minimized or dismissed, leaving us to feel *disenfranchised grief.* Dr. Kenneth Doka describes this as "grief that results when a person experiences a significant loss and the resultant grief is not openly acknowledged, socially validated, or publicly mourned."[3] Grief can be hard to bear, and more so if we feel like our loss is not valid and we have no right to grieve. Those of us grieving womb loss may feel this deeply given the prevailing stigma, shame, and even criminalization of certain forms of womb loss. But even if our grief is not widely understood or supported, we can choose to tend to our grief with our own internal resources, knowing for ourselves that our loss is real, our grief is valid, and that we have every right to mourn.

The following practice is an invitation to reflect on your fertility journey as a whole. Even when society does not see or acknowledge the value of your felt experience, you can know your own value as you realize all you have endured.

GROUNDING REFLECTION PRACTICE

Your Fertility Timeline

I often remind fellow womb loss survivors—be they loved ones or my postpartum doula clients—that their felt experience in this moment is a culmination of many experiences over the course of their fertility journey. They may not only be grieving their most recent womb loss but also others that came before. They may be grieving the months or years of trying to conceive only to feel disappointment each time their period began. They may be grieving their decision to hold off on trying to conceive because that's what their partner wanted or so they could focus on their education or career, even if they would not do it differently. Reflecting on the entirety of your fertility journey, including your losses, can help you cultivate compassion toward yourself for all you have gone through and also appreciation for your resilience in enduring so much. You will need paper and something to write with.

The Invitation

Taking your time, find a comfortable position before bringing your awareness to your breath. Allow your body to breathe naturally, maybe deepening your breath to help you feel more grounded in this moment. When you are ready, begin documenting your fertility timeline by writing down any memorable moments. This can be in chronological order, with or without dates, or simply a list of moments as they come to you intuitively. You might include moments like when you first got your period, when you became sexually active, if you were sexually assaulted, when you met your birth partner, when you decided to start a family without a partner, the times you have been pregnant, your expected due dates, when you were diagnosed with a health condition(s) that impacted your fertility, the times you experienced pregnancy or infant loss, your baby's/babies' birth date(s) and death date(s), when you held their funeral service, when you began fertility treatment, when you decided to stop trying to conceive. As you can see, there is much that can be written. There is so much we can go through. Acknowledge aspects of your fertility that are meaningful to you.

Once you have finished, sit a moment with what you've written, taking in all that landed on the page(s). Consider what you have experienced in your fertility journey thus far. How does it feel to look at this paper? How do you feel toward your body? When you feel ready to bring this practice to a close, you can take a deep cleansing breath, perhaps allowing the exhalation to be audible, or press down into the parts of you touching the earth. You have been through so much, dear reader. May you know this and that you deserve to be held in love.

Postpartum Champorado (Chocolate Rice Porridge)

A Recipe by Eileen S. Rosete

I recently cooked this recipe for my beloved friend Katrina on a very tender anniversary, the due date of one of her children and the death date of another. Her child, Zeo Thomas, would have been born that day had he not died in the womb at five months gestation. It was within the same year of his death that her second child, Solis Vida, died in the womb in the first trimester. In truth, Katrina had been bleeding for over a week to release her second pregnancy, but as she bled through Zeo's due date, she felt an intuitive pull to honor this same date as Solis's death date.

I thought of my friend as I made my way slowly through the grocery store. Though it was crowded and busy, I felt cocooned in my thoughts and intentions for her—how I wanted to help her feel seen and held during this difficult time—and I found myself gathering each of the ingredients in a mindful way that felt like the beginning of a bigger ritual. Knowing I was going to cook for her to honor her, her babies, her grief, and also her longings added a layer of reverence to what would otherwise be a standard grocery run. Later as I cooked the porridge in her home, I channeled my love and condolences into each step. And when I finally brought the warm bowl of champorado to her and saw her reaction, it was my turn to feel honored. Honored to be there with her. Honored to tend to her. And with a dish we both knew from our childhoods. She dubbed it "postpartum champorado," and so it shall be known.

~

Warm and soft, rice porridge is one of the best postpartum foods as it is easy to eat, warming to the body, and gentle on the digestive system. Its very nature is to offer comfort. In my opinion, champorado, a Filipino chocolate rice porridge I grew up savoring, is one of the most heartwarming dishes, with the cacao tending as much to the emotional heart as to the physical body. It can be offered any time of day for both a filling meal and a gentle reminder that there is still sweetness in life even amidst grief. In this nourishing version, cacao powder is used in place of cocoa so that we may benefit from all that this superfood has to offer, including iron to help rebuild red blood cells, flavonoids to improve blood flow, and magnesium to ease anxiety and depression. In addition to being nutrient-rich, cacao is also known to lift the mood.

If the thought of preparing food feels beyond your current capacity in this moment, consider sharing this recipe with a partner, postpartum doula, or other support person and asking them to cook it for you. Additionally, if you are currently pregnant, please consult your health-care provider before consuming cacao as it contains caffeine.

- 1 cup sweet rice (also called glutinous or sticky rice) or sushi rice

- 5 cups water

- 1/4 cup cacao powder

- 1/2 cup brown sugar

- 1 tablespoon unflavored protein powder (optional)

- Condensed coconut milk for topping

- Cacao nibs (optional)

Rinse the sweet rice several times until the water runs clear when drained. Combine rice and water in a pot over medium-high heat. Bring to a boil, then reduce heat to medium and continue to cook until the rice is soft and the porridge thickens (about 20 minutes), stirring often to keep from sticking to the bottom of the pot. Add cacao powder, brown sugar, and unflavored protein powder. Stir to combine, then remove from heat. Drizzle condensed coconut milk (or other milk of choice) and top with cacao nibs. Serve hot.

The Layers of Our Grief

Grief is so often a layered experience. We are not just grieving the *primary loss* of the ending of our pregnancy or the death of our baby, we are also often grieving multiple or many *secondary losses*—losses that flow from the primary loss. In womb loss, secondary losses may include loss of our role as a parent to that child, loss of our role as a parent to any or any more living children (secondary infertility), loss of health, loss of identity, loss of intimacy with our partner, loss of our partner, loss of hopes for the future, loss of self-worth, loss of our pre-pregnant body, loss of faith, loss of trust in our health-care providers, loss of finances. This is but a handful of secondary losses often felt in connection to womb loss. As they add up, secondary losses can compound an already overwhelming primary loss and deepen our grief.

Tending to your physical body when your emotional body is overwhelmed can help to soften both. The following practice invites you to offer gentle warmth to your postpartum womb. May it help ease all the layers of grief you embody.

GROUNDING EMBODIMENT PRACTICE

Warming the Womb

We all begin in the womb, feeling held within its comforting warmth as our needs are tended to with instinctual care. This practice of self-tending invites warmth to your own womb, helping it and you feel held. If making any kind of contact with this part of your body does not feel resonant for you, that is completely understandable and okay. The belly, the womb space, is such a tender place to begin with, and womb loss can make our relationship with it more complex. If you are unsure how you feel about making contact with your belly, perhaps follow the invitation and note any felt sensations that arise, knowing you can choose to stop at any time. Learning what feels comforting and healing for you can be a process. Honor what feels right to you in this moment. You will need a heating pad and a hand towel.

The Invitation

Prepare your heating pad following the appropriate directions for the type you are using and place a hand towel on your womb space to avoid any painful exposure to heat (or you can simply place it over a shirt you are wearing). Then, gently apply the heating pad to your belly, letting it rest here for as long as it feels okay. Alternatively, if you don't have access to a heating pad, you can dampen a hand towel with warm water, then squeeze to remove excess water before testing it on your skin to ensure the heat is comfortable. Once it is, gently drape it over your belly. You may find it helpful to sit in a reclined position or to lie down to help keep the towel in place. If you are acutely postpartum, warmth on the belly can help soothe any postpartum cramping (known as afterpains) as your womb continues to contract to return to its nonpregnant state over the course of about six weeks (known as uterine involution). If you are further along in your postpartum time and your periods have resumed, a heating pad can offer relief from menstrual cramps.[4] Perhaps consider applying a heating pad to other parts of your body, such as the neck and shoulders, allowing the warmth to sink in and melt away any tension. And if applying a heating pad feels supportive to your body, perhaps explore making this a daily or weekly ritual of self-tending that can help you wind down and ease into rest.

Honoring Your Grief

Remember, there is no right or wrong way to grieve. Gently remind yourself of this if you ever notice yourself thinking, "I *should* feel . . ." Grieving is feeling, and how you feel is entirely unique to you. That said, there are models and theories about grief that may offer insight into your own process and language to describe your felt experience. Should you refer to them, keep them in mind as suggestions or guidelines, integrating what resonates and leaving what doesn't. And as you grieve, know that while it is natural to compare your grief to the grief of others, grief truly cannot be compared. For example, it is common for those who experience early pregnancy loss to minimize their grief when they compare their loss to a stillbirth later in pregnancy. What your loss means to you and how you feel about it is what matters most. All grief deserves to be acknowledged. All grief deserves to be tended to with gentleness. All grief deserves to be honored.

The following practice is an invitation to connect with your body and the grief held within. May it support you in acknowledging and honoring your unique felt experience and grieving process.

A Letter to Your Body

For this practice, you will need a journal and two differently colored pens. Choose a new journal (or perhaps remove pages from an existing one) to dedicate to your grief, creating a sacred container you can pour into whenever your grief feels like too much to carry.

The Invitation

When you feel ready, find a quiet place and a comfortable seated position. In your own time, invite your awareness to gently focus on your in-breath and out-breath, allowing your body to soften with each exhalation and letting any other thoughts melt away. Perhaps soften your gaze or close your eyes and notice any sensations in your body. When it feels right, open your eyes if they are closed and reach for your journal and a pen. Take time now to write a letter to your body. Allow yourself to be honest and to express what you feel, even if it is hard to see it on paper. Once you have finished, turn the paper over and in a different color pen, write a letter from your body to you. Allow your body to have quality time and space to express itself to you. When this practice feels complete, you can close your journal with care and take a deep cleansing breath to gently mark your transition from this activity to the rest of your day.

Allow yourself compassion for all that may have arisen for you during this practice of connecting with your body and the grief it is carrying. It can be difficult to do if you live in a culture that does not model this. You may not realize you are worthy of such compassion if you do not see it clearly reflected in the world around you. In such cases, allow yourself to nurture loving-kindness toward your body as best you can, one caring act at a time.

You May Always Carry Your Grief

Just as there is no right or wrong way to grieve, there is no definitive timeline for grief. You may always carry your grief, and that's okay. The concept of *continuing bonds* that editors Dennis Klass, Phyllis Silverman, and Steven Nickman explore in their book *Continuing Bonds: New Understandings of Grief* validates that grief is ongoing, normal, and even helpful to stay connected to your loved one.[5] Your relationship with your pregnancy, with your baby, can in fact continue, albeit in a different way than you may have imagined. So rather than feel a pressure to "move on" or "get over it," know that you can instead maintain and nurture your connection throughout your life. Know, too, that how your grief feels may shift over time. It may not always feel as heavy and debilitating as it does at the start. Its intensity may soften even as its meaning deepens, becoming more of a warm connection, a tender presence. Honor the unique unfolding of your own grieving process, your feeling process, without feeling pressure to do it "right."

No matter where you are in your grieving and postpartum healing journey, no matter how intense or quiet your grief may be, know that you are worthy of feeling witnessed. The following practice invites you to ask another person to bear witness to you, to hold space for you with compassion. Feeling seen by another human being can be medicine when enduring womb loss. Remember, you are not alone, nor should you feel alone.

GROUNDING RELATIONAL PRACTICE

Ask for a Silent Witness

Learning what kind of support we need from others can be a process. We may not know what we need; therefore, we may not know what to ask. Or we may ask for something and then realize it wasn't actually helpful. Have courage to reach out for support and learn through experience what others can do to truly tend to your needs.

The Invitation

Practice asking someone you trust—such as a partner, a friend, or a family member—if they could spend some time with you as a silent witness. To silently sit with you, walk with you, lie next to you, ride bikes with you— however you want to spend your time with them. As they hold space for you in silence, allow yourself to share what you are thinking or feeling, or simply join them in the silence. You can use any of the following suggestions or other phrasing that feels right for you.

- Can you sit silently with me for a while?
- Can you sit silently with me while I share how I'm feeling?
- Could we go for a silent walk with the option for me to talk if it feels right?

As is often the case, those we turn to for support may not know what to do or say, or they may do or say something that feels insensitive to us despite their best intentions. This practice is one way you can feel supported while also deterring any such acts or comments. Asking for what you need is a practice. If it's hard or uncomfortable, that's okay. See if this changes the more you exercise your ability to name your needs.

Offering from the Collective

The following is an offering from a dear friend and my longtime acupuncturist, Michelle. We met in Chicago when I was pregnant for the first time over nine years ago, and she has tended to me through all of my pregnancies and all of my losses. Even after we moved to California, I made it a priority to see her every time we went back to the Midwest because her healing ability is that strong and her spirit that uplifting. My naps are the deepest when I am in her treatment room at the Raby Institute for Integrative Medicine, a beautiful sanctuary in the middle of downtown Chicago. With her, I feel so seen, so held, so safe. I invited Michelle to share the following offering so that you may know Traditional Chinese Medicine, acupuncture, and essential oils can be integrated into your own grieving and postpartum healing process. And so that you may feel how I feel when I am with her—loved.

Traditional Chinese Medicine, Acupuncture, and Essential Oils

What it is

Traditional Chinese Medicine (TCM) is an ancient healing art rooted in the belief that your body is an integrated whole that pulses vital life force energy (or qi, pronounced "chee") along channels called meridians. Beautifully complex, your physical body, mind, emotions, and spiritual being dance together to influence this delicately attuned energetic system. When these channels become obstructed or depleted, imbalances arise. Profound healing emerges when qi is restored to a balanced state. TCM modalities support this rebalancing and include acupuncture, acupressure, cupping, gua sha, herbal medicine, tuina, tai chi, qi gong, and dietary therapy.

Acupuncture, which has grown in popularity in Western medicine, has been widely studied and practiced for over five thousand years. Tiny needles, positioned at specific access points along meridians, promptly activate energy flow in the body. This activation calls forward a healing shift—one of mental, physical, emotional, or spiritual change.

Essential oils—extracted from florals, fruits, herbs, roots, and resins—are medicinal plant essences that carry unique molecules and energetic vibrations into the body through skin absorption or inhalation. Their powerful frequencies support activation of energy flow by way of the circulatory system and the olfactory nerve. These aromatic essences merge with the limbic system of the brain, which regulates our emotions, behavior, and memory, and can enrich healing at many levels. They can be used in several ways, including the following:

- Inhaled directly from an open bottle
- Added to and inhaled from diffuser jewelry

- Added to an essential oil diffuser, humidifier, or more simply to a napkin then inhaled

- Added to the shower walls to inhale as you shower

- Added to bath water after being diluted with a carrier oil (e.g., coconut, jojoba)

- Applied directly to skin (e.g., a few drops to the wrists or behind the neck or via massage) after being diluted with a carrier oil

How it can support you

One extraordinary meridian in TCM is the Bao Mai, or the Uterus Vessel. When accessed, this delicate channel supports nourishment between the heart and the womb and cultivates the deepest form of self-exploration. The heart houses the shen, which roughly translates as "spirit" or "presence of self." The womb translates to "moon or child palace." Activating and calling open this channel, tenderly, with acupuncture, breath, and/or essential oils can support spiritual and physiological healing from pregnancy or infant loss. Whether you are struggling with postpartum anxiety, depression, grief, digestive imbalances, abdominal or pelvic pain, circulation imbalances, TMJ, headaches, and more, you can benefit from this energetic awakening of the Bao Mai channel.

Bravely Softening and Strengthening the Bao Mai Channel

A self-tending practice

Our lungs, the delicate organs associated with grief in Eastern medicine, assist the energy of the heart to carry blood along the Bao Mai channel. Expanding our breath allows us to soften into grief and healing from loss.

1. To begin, find yourself in a comfortable and safe space for self-tending. Pause, become present with your breath, and take notice of your heart-womb vibration. Without judgment, let your intuition rise up to guide you.

2. Place one drop of rose, jasmine, or neroli essential oil in the palm of your hand with roughly one teaspoon of carrier oil (jojoba or coconut).

Rose, jasmine, and neroli oils soften the heart from trauma and are considered "heart hug" oils as they nurture and expand your capacity for self-love and tender care. They also support hormone regulation and rebalancing.

3. Rub your hands together gently, then cup both palms over your nose. Inhale and exhale the essence deeply, one to three times. Honor the quiet shift.

4. Gently apply the oil to the breastbone located between the nipples, acupoint Conception Vessel 17 (CV17). This point tonifies lung and heart energy and encourages emotional sturdiness. Use soft, downward strokes toward your womb to invite a smooth and open flow.

5. Peacefully sit or lie down. Close your eyes and place your left hand over your heart, and if it feels okay to do so, your right hand over your womb, holding yourself lovingly. Continue taking unrushed and nourishing breaths for as long as feels right, and visualize tending to your inner heart-womb garden—delicate, fragrant, wounded, resilient, and full of reverence. Whisper to yourself this sweet gift: *I deserve to be held and to heal.*

A Gentle Closing

Thank you for being here. For showing up for yourself, your body, and your grief as we explored grief in the context of womb loss. Grief is a natural response to a loss that is meaningful, and grief felt as a result of womb loss is as valid as any other. Grief is also layered, ever shifting, and even everlasting. May you be gentle with yourself as you tend to your grief. This can be as simple as asking yourself, "Where does it hurt?" Then listening to what your body has to share. Know, too, that you can turn to any of the grounding practices here and throughout the book for support.

As this chapter comes to a close, I invite you to pause for a few breaths and with the closing verse to help you transition gently back into your life or to the next part of the book. And if anything in this chapter activated a strong response, consider doing something more to feel grounded. This may be an act of self-tending or reaching out to someone you trust for support. Honor what you need in this moment.

I am here, as I am.
And so it is.

You are here.
And we are with you.

CHAPTER 5

When Grief and Trauma Intersect

You deserve to feel safe.

What I had thought would be a short tour of Great Vow Zen Monastery in Clatskanie, Oregon, unfolded into a full day of slow walking, warm conversations, and deep breaths of fresh country air. A sense of reverence permeated the grounds of this converted 1970s-era elementary school, mirroring what is naturally imbued in the ancient forest behind it. I had learned of the monastery and its cofounder Jan Chozen Bays in my research of grief rituals. A pediatrician specializing in the evaluation of child abuse, Zen teacher, and survivor of pregnancy loss, Chozen has been leading Jizo ceremonies for the past thirty years. In Buddhism, Jizo is regarded as a protector of travelers through the physical and spiritual realms including children who have died at any age, even before birth, and for any reason. As explained by Chozen, "Jizo has begun to fill a small but unique spiritual niche in America, honored as the central figure in ceremonies of remembrance for children who have died, in particular those lost through miscarriage and abortion."[1]

I was shown to the room where the Jizo ceremonies at Great Vow Monastery take place. I paused in awe as I took in the womb-like room, complete with a carpeted sunken circle seating area in the center. The air of reverence was certainly thicker here. I learned that attendees gather in this space and spend time making a simple toy, necklace, or small garment in honor of their child who died. Afterward, they walk outside to the Jizo

Bodhisattva remembrance garden where they are invited to leave their items on the Jizo statues that rest there. It is a very simple ceremony done in silence.

Though the room was empty while I was there, I could sense into the grief that attendees carried in. And later, as I walked into the remembrance garden, I could feel a noticeable difference between one side of the wooden threshold and the other where countless Jizos stood, silently holding space throughout the forest. Some new, some old, and some ancient, brought from Japan. Some clothed in moss, others in items left from ceremonies past. It is a place of whispers and careful steps. And very deep sadness.

Later, after lunch, I sat with Chozen in the dining hall—just the two of us in the afternoon shadows. I looked into the eyes of this elder who had witnessed and held space for so much pain. For so long. And who carried her own felt experience of womb loss. I listened to her wisdom, to stories of her work with the bereaved. I will end here with one such story.

Chozen described to me a woman she had met in Japan. A bereaved mother who each year placed a food offering at her child's altar. She never offered the same thing. Instead, the food changed as the mother imagined what she would have fed her child at that age had her child lived.

This story brought tears to my eyes and my right hand to my heart as it ached for this mother. I saw my tears reflected in Chozen's eyes. Initially, I was surprised to see her tear up. I suppose the thought that she had held space for pregnancy and infant loss for decades and that her own losses were just as far past led me to think she would not be as affected by the story. But as we sat in silence for a long moment, simply gazing into each other's tears, I was reminded that the trauma of womb loss can leave lasting imprints on our being. I was honored to bear witness to Chozen's show of emotion and to feel such deep connection in our shared grief despite the many years separating us and our losses. Both of us, bereaved mothers, knew the kind of pain the mother in her story felt—that deep longing to want to care for our children who died.

~

As you will be reminded many times over, you are not alone, dear reader. Across continents and generations, womb loss and the trauma that can accompany it have been felt, are being felt, and will continue to be felt. We are hurting with you. And we are hurting for you.

Understanding Trauma

Trauma is a deep impression that makes it difficult to feel safe and at ease. It can be caused by a single, painful event that we experience ourselves or witness, or it can result from an accumulation of events, such as coping with systemic issues like sexism and racism on a regular basis. Such impressions have the power to influence how we think, feel, and act. Trauma can also be inherited if left untended, as it influences the lived experiences of one generation and is then felt by the following generation(s). But even such deep and lasting impressions can soften when we acknowledge and tend to them with care.

Womb loss is an experience that feels deeply traumatic for many and can be referred to as a form of *birth trauma, reproductive trauma,* or *pregnancy loss trauma.* I also resonate with Dr. Peter Levine's definition: "Trauma is not what happens to us. But what we hold inside in the absence of an empathetic witness."[2] Birth trauma is, as the name implies, trauma rooted in a birth experience. The March of Dimes defines it as "any physical or emotional distress you may experience during or after childbirth."[3] Up to 45 percent of new moms experience birth trauma. In the context of womb loss, I would add that such distress can be experienced before birth when we first learn about our loss. Trauma can severely affect our behaviors and emotions as we try to find ways to cope with it, so it is essential to tend to our trauma just as we tend to our grief and postpartum needs. Healing after womb loss is layered this way. Remember, you are not alone as you tend to these layers.

The following practice is an invitation to tend to the trauma you carry. It encourages gentle self-touch and diaphragmatic breathing, which initiates our rest-and-digest state and helps our body feel safe to soften. Please move with care. Notice how it feels to bring your hands to the sides of your front body. If placing your hands so close to your womb space causes discomfort, that is okay. You can rest your hands in your lap instead and direct your breath to your diaphragm without touch.

Self-Hug Breathing

Improving the quality of your breath can improve your entire well-being. The following practice engages your diaphragm when breathing to help you relax and ease stress and anxiety.

The Invitation

Taking your time, find your way into a comfortable seated position before allowing your awareness to follow your breath. Then, if it feels okay, you are welcome to cross your arms in front of your chest, placing your palms at the sides of your ribs. Allow your breath to flow to the areas directly below your hands, helping to improve the quality of your breathing. Allow yourself to feel held as you hold yourself in a warm, compassionate hug. Perhaps explore closing your eyes or softening your gaze as you breathe here for as long as it feels right to you. When you are ready to bring this practice of grounding and self-tending to a close, take a deep cleansing breath or press into the parts of you that are touching the earth and slowly open your eyes if they are closed.

You deserve respectful, gentle touch such as this. Even from yourself. Especially from yourself. You can do something as simple as giving yourself a hug to nurture a felt experience of being held and loved, and to counter the trauma you feel.

Trauma and Our Postpartum Body

Trauma affects everyone differently. Birth trauma, like womb loss, is unique given that our bodies are the site of the event(s) we experienced as traumatic. So, we may harbor feelings of distrust or betrayal toward our bodies. Our body may not feel like a safe or comfortable place because of the trauma we carry, the grief we carry, and all the changes our body has experienced through pregnancy and birth. With such internal discord, it may take a great deal of effort to simply exist in our bodies, much less understand its cues and tend to its needs. If your relationship with your body feels challenging in the midst of and after womb loss, that is understandable, and it is okay.

The following is an invitation to nurture a gentle connection with your body. In moments of struggle when your trauma is activated and you find yourself unable to cope, it can be hard to think of what to do to help yourself or what to ask of others. Creating a comfort kit for such moments can offer both you and your loved ones the reassurance that there are practical tools within reach.

GROUNDING MINDFULNESS PRACTICE

Create a Comfort Kit

For this practice, you will need a container (a box, a bag, a basket, etc.) and items that help you feel safe, grounded, and at ease.

Ideas for Comfort Kit Items

The items included in a comfort kit will look different for each person. Choose items that can help you feel grounded in moments when you feel your trauma being activated. These can be items that help your mind focus on an object through touch and sight, items that allow your mind a safe distraction (such as a calming or pleasurable book, or photos that bring a smile to your face), items that help you externalize what you are feeling in a creative way (such as art supplies), items that invite gentle movement, items that allow your mind to focus on your sense of taste (such as a snack), and items that are soft and comforting to touch. These might be items you have used in the past, or they may be new. Know that you can try items and switch them out at any time. Here is a list of ideas to help as you decide what honors your needs.

- Blank journal
- Coloring book
- Pen
- Colored pencils
- Comforting photos
- Book

- Essential-oil body mist or room spray
- Essential-oil roller
- Aromatherapy lotion
- Snacks
- Eye pillow
- Stress ball or squishy toy
- Crochet or knitting supplies, or simply yarn for finger knitting
- Rose quartz stone (rose quartz is associated with self-love)
- Heating pad
- Shawl or blanket

The Invitation

Take some time today or gradually over the course of the week to gather items for your personal comfort kit. As you think of items to include, you might imagine what it would be like to use it and see how this lands in your body. Does it inspire a sense of comfort or relief? You might decide to take longer to create your comfort kit, and that is okay too. Honor your pace. You might also find that your needs shift; you can update your comfort kit at any point.

Once you've gathered all the items you would like, assemble them in your kit in a quiet moment, or you might consider putting them into your container with a greater sense of ritual and reverence. If the latter resonates with you, find a quiet place where you can be alone without interruption. You might explore creating a more soothing environment by turning on music that feels peaceful to you and even lighting a candle. Or you might find a moment alone outdoors, maybe laying a blanket on the earth for you to rest on, allowing the power of Mother Nature to support you as you assemble your comfort kit.

1. Find a comfortable seated position and have your comfort kit container and items within reach. You might notice the grounding sensation of the earth below your feet or sit bones; perhaps explore a gentle rocking motion side to side to actively ground and connect with the earth's energy. Allow yourself to feel held.

2. Then, taking your time, take a few deep breaths to activate your rest-and-relaxation state, allowing yourself to sink into this moment. You might even close your eyes or soften your gaze.

3. When you are ready, open your eyes if they are closed and begin to slowly, mindfully, take one item at a time into your hand, noticing how it looks and feels. You might offer an intention silently or aloud as you hold each item, such as, *Please help me to feel at ease.*

4. Then, take a conscious breath as you place it in your container. Once you have placed all the items in your container, close your eyes or soften your gaze and bring your palms to touch at your heart center or rest your hands over your heart. If it feels right, take a few deep breaths as you consider one word that encompasses how you feel in this moment. All of you is welcome here, so feel free to acknowledge whatever word emerges, either silently or aloud. There is no right or wrong way to feel.

5. When you are ready to bring this practice to a close, take a deep cleansing breath or press into the parts of you touching the earth and slowly open your eyes if they are closed.

Consider finding a place for your comfort kit that is easily accessible to you and also to your loved ones so that they can bring it or items from it to you when you ask or they notice you are experiencing a difficult moment. Remember, it is okay to state your needs, and it is okay to ask others to help meet your needs. If it feels right, you might consider making multiple comfort kits, such as one for your home and one to take when you are on the go or to leave in your car or at your workplace.

Softening Our Transitions

When we experience sudden, shocking, and traumatic transitions like womb loss, it can help to exercise our sovereignty by choosing to soften our daily transitions. Softening is self-tending, and you deserve to feel connected to your agency and ability to choose. Softening our transitions may look like:

- Moving slowly

- Simplifying our schedules

- Allowing more time and breathing room between one activity and the next

- Establishing a daily rhythm that infuses our days with a feeling of consistency and structure

- Having rituals to start and end our days

- Asking for help if doing so helps us feel more at ease

- Taking deep breaths before moving on

When you carry trauma, your body does its best to protect you from further harm by staying alert and ready to act—a constant state of hypervigilance that can be exhausting. Softening requires a sense of safety. To soften, we can nurture a sense of safety within ourselves. The following practice is an invitation to tend to your trauma so that you can feel safer to soften in moments throughout your day.

GROUNDING REFLECTION PRACTICE

A Memory of Safety

For this practice you will need paper and something to write with.

The Invitation

Find your way into a comfortable seated position and take a moment to connect with your breath. When you are ready, think of a time when you felt safe, when you felt so safe your body softened. Allow a distinct memory to emerge naturally. Describe this memory on paper with words or drawings. Do so from an embodied place, feeling the comfort you felt then filling your body once more. In trauma, it can feel hard to access a sense of safety. Know that this memory and the felt experience it offers are available to you any time. When you are ready to bring this practice to a close, take three deep breaths to soften your transition back into your space, back into your life.

Soothing Salt Bath Recipe

Trauma can manifest in our body as clenched muscles, constriction of the throat, chronic aches and pain, and migraines. The following is a simple salt bath recipe to help tend to these issues. This recipe offers the combined healing power of Epsom salt, which is widely used to relax muscles, and vanilla, a warm, sweet scent that is highly regarded for its ability to encourage relaxation, ease anxiety and depression, and lift our mood.

- 1 cup Epsom salt
- 2 tablespoons carrier oil (sweet almond, jojoba, or coconut oil)
- 4–6 drops of vanilla essential oil or oil of your choice that is safe for contact with the skin

Combine salt, carrier oil, and essential oil in a bowl or jar and mix. Run a warm to hot bath (consult with your health-care provider to ensure it is safe for you to take a bath depending on how recently you gave birth) and pour in the contents of the bowl. As you rest in the water, allow yourself to soften and be held. May you feel a sense of safety here.

Honoring Strong Feelings

It is common for survivors of womb loss to experience a spectrum of intense emotions, including anger, guilt, and shame. Anger about the outcome and the support we did or did not receive. Guilt about what we might have done differently, even if the loss could not be prevented. Shame about our bodies and how they could not function the way we wanted, the way society expects them to. These are big, intense feelings to carry within us, and they can make it challenging to be kind to ourselves and our bodies. Feelings are neither inherently good nor bad, though some may be harder to bear than others. It may help to think of feelings as a way our body communicates with us. Imagine each feeling as a distinct part of you. What is each feeling trying to tell you? What needs is each feeling trying to bring your attention to? In chapter 3, you were invited to identify feeling words.

Perhaps return to the words that resonated with you. For example, if you circled the word *anxious,* you could consider the part of you that feels anxious and ask it, "What do you need in this moment?" You might also think of feelings in terms of energy. Whenever you have big feelings, it can be hard to hold all that energy in your body, so you might find ways to soften and even release it. This can include some kind of physical movement, which can range from subtle and gentle to bigger and more rigorous. For example, doing yoga, walking, dancing, singing, screaming, or crying. Allow yourself to explore options to see what helps you.

The following practice invites you to engage in gentle physical activity to connect with your body and metabolize any big feelings.

GROUNDING EMBODIMENT PRACTICE

Counting Each Step

The Invitation

Take a walk, outdoors if possible, and count your steps. Allow the act of counting to be an anchor for your mind to hold on to, especially if your thoughts are racing, your breathing is shallow, or you are feeling overwhelmed in any way. As you walk, allow your body to generate a gentle heat within to help metabolize whatever you are holding on to. You can imagine whatever feels hard or heavy to carry leaving your body as you sweat and exhale. If your mind wanders, that's okay. Invite your awareness back to counting each step (picking up where you left off or starting your count again), or release the counting and walk in a way that feels right for you. Perhaps listening with a gentle awareness to the sounds around you or to music. Change your pace or come to rest whenever you desire. You are in full control here. Honor what you need.

Softer Self-Talk

Words are powerful, and talking to ourselves with compassion is essential to both our grieving and our healing. At the beginning of this book, we talked about the need for a softer shared language as we name our experiences, as we interact with health-care providers and birth workers, and as we talk with other womb loss survivors. It is essential that a softer language exist within us too, that our inner voice or self-talk is grounded in compassion. If you have ever been to a trauma-informed yoga class, you may have noticed the stark difference in language used by the instructor. In typical yoga classes, we are accusomed to being told what to do and how to feel: "From Tadasana, reach your arms up, lower the shoulders, and press strongly into your feet for Urdhva Hastasana. Feel how it energizes your body." In a trauma-informed yoga class, you will hear language that *invites* you to make choices that honor your needs and notice your unique experience: "When you are ready, you might reach your arms up as you allow your shoulders to melt down. And if it feels okay, you might explore pressing your feet into the earth as you come into Urdhva Hastasana. Notice how this feels for your body and make any adjustments you need to feel safe." Hearing such invitational language in class has often led me to tear up. You deserve to feel the comfort of softer, gentler language. Know that this is something you can offer yourself.

The following practice is an invitation to nurture softer self-talk so that your internal landscape can be a kinder place to be.

GROUNDING RITUAL PRACTICE

Gentle Reframes

For this practice you will need paper and something to write with.

The Invitation

Taking your time, find your way into a comfortable seated position. You might light a candle to mark the beginning of this practice and invite a feeling of reverence. Then, allow your awareness to follow your breath, perhaps deepening the breath to help you feel more grounded in this moment. When you are ready, draw a line down the middle of your paper or fold it in half, and on one side write the statements you've said to yourself that are more critical or negative in nature. On the opposite side of the line or fold of the paper, rephrase the sentence from a place of compassion. For example, on the left side I would write, "I should have started trying to conceive sooner," and on the right side I would write, "I wanted to start a family, *and* it was important to me to finish school. I made the best decision I could at the time." Continue doing this for as long as it feels right to you—writing critical statements on one side and gentle reframes on the other. When you are ready to bring this practice to a close, you are welcome to place one or both hands over your heart as you read aloud all the gentle reframes. Allow the softness of your own words to embrace you and allow the gentle pressure of your hands over your heart to warm you. Take a few deep breaths or press into the parts of you touching the earth, and blow out the candle.

Exercising Choice

In healing from trauma, especially trauma like womb loss that is so intimately connected to your own body, it can be incredibly helpful to connect with your agency by making choices for yourself. Doing so can help ease the pain of feeling utterly powerless in situations like womb loss. Accessing your agency can look like naming your needs and setting boundaries that you believe will help you feel safe. Even the most seemingly small decisions can be meaningful, and the culmination of many choices can go a long way toward rebuilding your confidence in yourself. The following practice invites you to exercise making choices and setting boundaries that help you center yourself and honor your needs.

GROUNDING RELATIONAL PRACTICE

A Self-Tending Mug

The following is inspired by Kimberly Ann Johnson, creator of The Fourth Trimester Cards. While she suggests reserving a bowl just for your own use, I invite you to choose a mug that can support you in tending to one of your most basic needs: hydration. For this practice you will need a mug (or a cup or a jar).

Choose a mug and designate it as *your* mug. No one else can use it except you. This could be a mug you already have or a new one you pick out intentionally for yourself and this practice. Choose one in a size, shape, color, or material that inspires a feeling of comfort, something you can come home to when you are in need of solace. You can also choose one that is beautiful to you and allow its beauty to lift your spirit each time you see it. Let your intuition guide you as you exercise choice in this simple though no less meaningful way.

The Invitation

Once you have chosen your mug, I invite you to infuse it with the intention of honoring you, your body, and your needs—perhaps by holding it, closing your eyes, and saying your intention silently or aloud. Next, let your loved ones know, whether verbally or perhaps by taping a note to it, that this is your mug. This is a chance for you to practice setting boundaries and clarifying expectations. Both are skills that can support your healing from trauma. Use your mug for any of the recipes shared here, water, or other drinks that honor your body's well-being. Let the daily practice of hydrating become a sacred act of self-tending.

Offering from the Collective

The following is an offering from a beloved friend, bereaved mother, and leading advocate for trauma-informed yoga. As I considered what healing modalities to highlight, trauma-informed yoga (also known as trauma-sensitive yoga) was top of mind. I know from personal experience that it can be an incredibly powerful modality not only for fitness but also for healing physically, emotionally, and spiritually. I reached out to Zabie so that you, dear reader, can know the power of trauma-informed yoga to reconnect you to your innate resilience, your power to choose, and your ability to heal on your own terms and in your own time.

Trauma-Informed Yoga

What it is

Trauma-informed yoga is an empowering yoga practice that centers the lived experience of each survivor as it invites integration of the mind, body, and spirit amidst the disintegration trauma causes. Safety, trust, choice, and control are some of the core components of the practice, and students are encouraged to honor their own pace and needs at all times. This is done through invitational language, supportive presence and co-regulation, sensitivity and support for triggers that might arise, offering variations for postures, creating accessibility for all bodies, trauma-sensitive breathwork, and integrating choice and consent throughout class.

How it can support you

Trauma-informed yoga can support survivors of womb loss in offering themselves the tenderness, care, and gentleness they deserve. The practice is designed to meet survivors where they are and support them in tending to physiological symptoms with care, enhancing their overall health, well-being, and resilience. The practice often helps survivors build incremental shifts over time to widen their window of tolerance, strengthen their coping skills, feel affirmed and seen, and, most importantly, feel empowered in their choices and grounded in their worth. This can ultimately lead to a space where survivors of womb loss can take powerful steps toward post-traumatic growth. Trauma-informed yoga can be a gentle and powerful way to reconnect with your body, even when and especially if you find it difficult to be in your body after womb loss. It can help you rebuild your connection to and trust in your body.

The following two self-tending practices are ones I hold near and dear to my heart. They have offered me comfort and gentle connection to my body as I grieved and continue to grieve a stillbirth at twenty-six weeks and a miscarriage at six weeks. I share them here with the hope that they help you in your grieving and healing process. Please know you are not alone in your pain and longing. You are held and supported by the love and understanding of so many. You are deeply seen and cherished.

Sun Meditation to Thaw Grief

A self-tending practice

I invite you to find a comfortable shape, sitting outside or inside where you can feel a sliver of sun. You might explore releasing your shoulders up and back and down, and invite your attention to the feeling of the sun on any parts of the body that need extra care and support. Perhaps you would like to rest your palms over your womb space if that feels supportive to you here. You might even envision that the sun is helping to soften and thaw any areas where trauma or grief might be held. Perhaps explore turning the volume of your heart up and the volume of your thoughts down. Everything you are feeling is valid and welcome in this space. Honor what might be coming to the surface, and be gentle with your experience. Take all the time you need, beloved; there is no rush.

Compassionate Face Cradle

A self-tending practice

When you feel ready, explore a seated shape that offers you a sense of safety and ease. Take all the time you need to set up, and use as many props as you can access to increase your comfort. If you'd like, begin to rub your palms together, creating a little bit of warmth. Whenever it feels right for you, gently rest your palms over your heart to take in your own care and compassion. You might explore a gentle rocking motion from side to side or front to back. Find a supportive and gentle rhythm and cadence that feel nurturing and accessible to you. When you are ready, you might bring your right hand to your right cheek and gently cradle it. You can continue the rocking motion if that feels supportive, and switch sides whenever you would like. Offer yourself your own compassion and care, and find any variation of this shape that honors what you need in this moment. Take all the time you need to find grounding in your own worthiness. Allow being where you are to be enough. It is enough.

Reminders for your practice:

- Send yourself gratitude just for arriving today. So often that is the hardest part.

- Take a moment to reflect on your journey and how far you've come. You are held and supported through it all.

- Today, explore taking up all the space you deserve.

- All parts of you are welcome here.

- Your choices are celebrated.

- You are worthy of gentleness and care.

A Gentle Closing

Thank you for being here. For showing up for yourself, your body, and your grief as we explored the intersection of grief and trauma in the context of womb loss. Our feelings of grief can be that much heavier when layered with trauma, with deep impressions that make it hard to feel safe, at ease, and show up for our lives the way we want. May you be gentle with yourself as you tend to the part of you that feels traumatized, knowing that your compassionate presence can do much to ease the pain. For you deserve to feel safe, now and always.

As this chapter comes to a close, I invite you to pause for a few breaths and with the closing verse to help you transition gently back into your life or to the next part of the book. And if anything in this chapter activated a strong response, consider doing something more to feel grounded. This may be an act of self-tending or reaching out to someone you trust for support. Honor what you need in this moment.

I am here, as I am.
And so it is.

You are here.
And we are with you.

CHAPTER 6

Our Loved Ones and Their Grief

What is yours to hold?

Evening shadows stretched into the dining room of my friend Joelle's home as my family and I headed toward the front door saying our goodbyes. We had just enjoyed a delicious home-cooked meal, laughter, and much longed for adult conversation while our living children played together. It was a wonderful reprieve after the long drive from Southern California to Calgary, Alberta, Canada on Moh'kinsstis Treaty 7 territory. We had arrived the day before, just in time to join Joelle and her family for the second annual Legacy Run/Walk hosted by the Pregnancy and Infant Loss Support Centre (PILSC) and to honor the recent birthday of their deceased son, Julien Wayne, who died in utero at six months gestation.

To walk with our partners and living children alongside so many others who knew womb loss as personally as we did was a deeply meaningful moment. I watched as a couple walked by with a double stroller—a living child in one seat and a teddy bear, a placeholder, in the other. I saw a large group of people wearing matching shirts with the name of the baby who died on the back and another group whose matching shirts said, "Held for a moment/Loved for a lifetime." I listened as local Indigenous healer and bereaved parent Daisy Giroux honored the land and shared plant medicine. Before burning sage and sweetgrass, she explained that sweetgrass is used for purification after experiences of struggle, and she invited us to join her in smudging ourselves. Later, I offered condolences to Joelle's mother, who was grieving the death of her second grandchild. As I walked, I took in the signs placed all along the route, including one that said, "Even those that never fully blossom bring beauty into the world." The energy at the park that morning was one of reverence, tempered sorrow, and tenderness, with a pervading sense of compassion as we gathered to honor our personal experiences of womb loss without the burden of judgment. There was a sense of intimacy despite the crowd as we collectively acknowledged our shared grief and mourned together by running, walking, and also fundraising. Through our joint efforts, we raised over $100,000.00 for the charity organization, which offers free support services accessible to people around the world.

Back in Joelle's home, I was almost to the front door when Joelle's husband, Calvin, turned to me and asked if I would like to light incense for our babies. I was stunned for a moment, caught off guard by his thoughtful offer. I said yes and watched as he invited my second living child to choose incense for their altar. I smiled as I heard the voice of their living son, Axel. He wanted to choose the incense stick, but as his parents explained, Vera would choose this time since she was their guest. Calvin then guided us to their family altar in the living room where my three living children looked on curiously and asked questions about the items displayed. Among them was Julien's tiny, beautiful blue urn resting atop his grandfather's larger rectangular one. The candles on the altar offered a soft glow, made more pronounced by the ever-darkening sky, as our families stood in silence for a moment to acknowledge our pregnancy losses and the babies we could not hold.

~

You are not alone, dear reader. There are many of us who know the pain of womb loss in our bodies and many who know the pain of womb loss alongside us. Know that we and our loved ones can grieve in our own unique ways while also grieving together. We can express our grief outwardly, mourning in our unique ways *and* mourning together. In the tender moment described above, we all stood in front of the beautiful altar participating in a simple and deeply meaningful ritual of remembrance. We mourned together as we simultaneously felt our unique internal experience of grief. Understanding that how we grieve and mourn may differ from how our loved ones grieve and mourn can help soften any feelings of isolation. We are in this process of grieving and healing together, though we may be moving through it differently and at our own pace. Honoring our own grief as we try to honor and support our loved ones' grief is a process that asks for gentle tending.

Sharing the News

Sharing your story of womb loss can be incredibly cathartic, and at the same time, whether or not you share the news of your womb loss is a highly personal decision. On one hand, it can be helpful to share and receive emotional and practical support in return. On the other hand, you may prefer to have privacy so you can focus on yourself rather than face others and their reactions. If you live somewhere that is not compassionate to your experience of womb loss, you may feel safer not sharing at all. You may also decide not to share the news now and then change your mind later. It may feel like enough to see others share their stories of womb loss, and that is okay too. According to therapist Nicole Makowka, LMFT, who co-led a miscarriage support group I participated in: "The sharing of perinatal loss experiences on social media really normalizes an experience that used to feel incredibly shameful. And it can be incredibly cathartic to sometimes just be an observer to someone else who's ready to share their story, because not only does it model some language around how to share a story, but it also normalizes a lot of feelings. It's that piece of permission that really goes missing when we as a society determine there are things that we can and can't talk about in public."[1]

If you are unsure what to do, you might take a moment to imagine sharing the news with someone in particular and notice how your body responds. Do you feel a sense of relief or notice your shoulders softening down? Do you feel a sense of anxiety or a tightening in your chest? Do you feel indifferent, with no noticeable physical response? There is no right or wrong decision. What matters most is what is meaningful to you.

It can be hard to share what we feel if the feelings are so big that they overwhelm us. The following practice invites you to use your breath to soften big feelings so you feel more able to be with them. If you are partnered or have living children, this practice can be done together and nurture healing connection amidst your shared loss. It is a practice that can work well for grievers of all ages and can be especially appealing to young children given its tactile nature. Sharing this practice can be a way to grieve together and cultivate a sense of comforting togetherness.

GROUNDING BREATHING PRACTICE

Hand-Tracing Breath

Part of the power of this widely practiced breathing exercise is its subtlety. You can turn to it anytime without drawing attention to yourself. It can prove especially useful in those in-between moments when you're waiting. Waiting for public transportation, waiting for the red light to turn green, waiting for your coffee order to be ready. You can allow those in-between moments to be a chance for self-tending. Part of the power of this practice is also in the act of gentle touch. When keeping your awareness on your breath is hard to do, adding an element of gentle, caring touch can offer your mind a physical sensation to follow, an external movement to watch and use as an anchor.

The Invitation

When you are ready, hold one hand up or place it on your lap. With a finger from the other hand, trace up the outside length of your thumb as you inhale through the nose and trace down the other side as you exhale through the mouth. Trace up the side of the next finger as you inhale through the nose and trace down the side of the finger as you exhale through the mouth. Continue tracing your fingers, and once you've traced up and down the pinky finger, you are welcome to stop there and switch hands or go in reverse to return to your thumb before switching hands.

If doing this with young living children, you might say, "If you ever have big feelings that are hard to hold inside, you can trace your hand like this and help those feelings become smaller." Then demonstrate by asking them to hold a hand up and invite them to breathe in with you as you gently trace up one side of a finger and breathe out as you gently trace down the other side.

Our Loved Ones and Their Grief   133

This may tickle, and you may share laughter with them. That is okay and even welcome. Grieving does not mean you must always feel sad (or any other emotion), and allowing for moments of laughter and levity doesn't mean your grief is any less real or any less deep. It is okay to feel moments of ease and even joy. It is okay to continue living.

Grieving Together and Differently

Even though our loved ones did not carry the pregnancy and in turn do not feel the loss in the same embodied way we do, they are still grieving the loss and processing what it means to them. So while it is important to center our bodies, our needs, and our grief, it is also important to honor that our loved ones are grieving too. In their own way. In their own time. And just as your grieving and healing process may be unfolding, so too may theirs. They may still be learning what it means to grieve and figuring out what support they need. What we do share with our loved ones is the truth that grieving is a full-being experience, and we all need tools to help us cope with the big feelings or strong sensations that arise. This includes love. Love for ourselves. Love for those grieving with us. It can be helpful to grieve together so we can feel the love we share and feel less alone. Grieving together can look many different ways. It can be honoring the loss through a shared act of mourning. It can simply be time spent together without bringing up the loss. As we honor our shared grief, it's important to recognize that each of us experiences and expresses our grief differently. And that is okay.

Underlying both grieving and healing from womb loss is loving-kindness. Loving-kindness for yourself. Your body. Your needs. Your grief. Offering yourself the very care you are worthy of receiving from others. And offering others the care they are worthy of receiving as well. The following practice is an invitation to offer yourself and others loving-kindness. You might consider returning to this practice whenever you are experiencing difficult moments with those who are grieving alongside you but differently.

A Loving-Kindness Meditation for Womb Loss

The Invitation

I welcome you to find a comfortable resting position seated or lying down. If seated, perhaps sit at the edge of a chair or on the front edge of a folded blanket to support a lengthening through the spine. If lying down, consider bending the knees and planting the soles of the feet on the earth to support the low back. Once you feel settled, begin by allowing your awareness to follow the gentle flow of your breath moving in and moving out of your body. Then allow your gaze to soften or your eyes to close. When you are ready, send loving-kindness to yourself with the following phrases, either silently or aloud:

May I feel seen,
May I feel heard,
May I feel held,
May I feel loved.

When you are ready, call to mind somebody else who has been affected by womb loss, saying their name either silently or aloud and perhaps picturing them in your mind's eye as you direct these phrases of loving-kindness to them:

May you feel seen,
May you feel heard,
May you feel held,
May you feel loved.

Finally, when you are ready, call to mind the collective of womb loss survivors—past, present, and future—as well as those who endured womb loss alongside them. Perhaps nurture an energetic connection to the collective as you offer these phrases of loving-kindness:

May we feel seen,
May we feel heard,
May we feel held,
May we feel loved.

Honoring Our Partner's Grief

It can be both challenging and important to honor our partner's grief as much as we honor our own. As mentioned throughout the book, grief and grieving are different for everyone. So while you and your partner may be grieving the same loss, how that grief feels for each of you and how you show it can be very different. These differences can lead to partners feeling disconnected, not on the same page, or even abandoned. One partner (often those of us who experience the loss with our body) may feel as if the loss means more to them, and they may feel hurt that their partner is not as affected. This can be due in part to the attachment we commonly begin to form with the pregnancy, with our baby, as soon as we learn we are pregnant and the subsequent decisions we make to protect our pregnancy (such as the foods we eat and the activities we do); whereas our partner may feel a stronger connection after we give birth when they can actually see and touch the baby. Among heterosexual couples, this can also be due in part to gender stereotypes that allow women expressing their emotions but discourage men from doing the same. May knowing it is common and okay for couples to respond to womb loss differently help to ease any tension in your relationship.

The following practice is an invitation to reflect on your partnership, if you are partnered, and what aspects you would like to carry into the days, weeks, months, and years ahead as you grieve and heal together.

GROUNDING REFLECTION PRACTICE

What Do You Want to Bring with You?

It can be helpful to reflect on how far your relationship with your partner has come as you bear your womb loss and to see what strengths your relationship can offer during this time of need. For this practice you will need paper and something to write with.

The Invitation

Find a quiet space and time to sit with each other. Create three columns on the paper by drawing two lines or folding the paper. Then begin to reflect on the strengths and growing edges (areas of difficulty) in your relationship before your womb loss and note these in the left column. Next, reflect on the strengths and growing edges in your relationship during your womb loss for the middle column. Finally, reflect on the strengths and growing edges in your relationship after your womb loss for the right column. Afterward, take a moment to see what landed on the page and reflect together. Are there any consistencies across the columns? Any significant shifts? Taking your time, turn the paper over and write down anything from the first three columns that you would like to bring into your relationship going forward. What would you want to experience again or more of? Perhaps place this paper somewhere you both can see it on a regular basis and allow it to be a gentle reminder of what your relationship is capable of.

Self-Tending Sugar Scrub Recipe

It can be difficult to feel at home in your body when you have experienced a trauma as intimate as womb loss. It can help to tend to your body in gentle and caring ways, slowly building a relationship with your body that feels safe. I share the following recipe with the memory of one of my own womb losses in mind. Immediately after giving birth, I made my way back into a hot shower and intuitively reached for the sugar scrub a friend had made. As I slowly and gently rubbed it on my body in circles and inhaled the sweet scent, I felt held in love, both by the tender touch I offered my body and by the spirit of my friend, whose loving intention I could feel from the product.

- Bowl
- 1 cup sugar
- 1/4 cup melted coconut oil

Add ingredients to the bowl and stir. Use by taking a small amount in hand while in a bath or shower and rub gently over your skin, then rinse with water.

Honoring Our Living Children's Grief

If you have living children, it is essential to acknowledge and honor that they are grieving too. Like you, they are trying to make sense of the loss and what it means. Like you, they may have big feelings that are hard to carry inside their bodies. While it is normal to include children in the preparations for a baby's arrival, in a grief-avoidant culture like the one we have in the US, we do not often include them if the pregnancy ends in loss. It is important to include surviving siblings in memorializing the loss and to give them opportunities to ask questions and share how they feel. We can help shift the culture around womb loss by helping younger generations know it as a common part of childbearing, as valid a loss as any other that deserves to be grieved. Additionally, we may think we need to be "strong" for our living children and equate "strong" with showing little to no emotion. But in fact, modeling grief as a natural response to loss and showing examples of how to grieve are essential life skills that can serve them whenever they experience a death. As you honor their unique experience of grief, trust too in their innate resilience.

The following practice is an invitation to engage in a gentle activity with those grieving alongside you and to feel the healing power of community.

GROUNDING EMBODIMENT PRACTICE

A Silent Walk

Silence has a way of quieting our minds and in turn easing our anxiety, heightening our awareness and also cultivating a sense of intimacy with ourselves and those with us. A silent walk can be a chance for you and your loved ones to spend quality time together without distractions and with more attentiveness to one another. It is essentially a form of witnessing, being with one another and with what is without trying to change anything. You might be more aware of one another's mood, body language, facial expressions than you normally would. You might notice things outdoors that you wouldn't if you had music or a podcast playing. You might notice details about yourself, your body, your grief that you hadn't before. Silence can help you realize what is essential.

The Invitation

Go for a silent walk outdoors with any loved ones who are grieving your loss with you (no talking, no music, etc.). This may include a partner, living children, or your parents. If you are within a year of birthing your loss, consider going for a slow walk as there may still be relaxin in your body causing your ligaments and joints to be loose.[2] How far you walk or how long you walk is completely up to you. If you have living children who are young, you might ask them to walk quietly while knowing it is in their nature to want to express themselves and share things with you. You might engage them in an activity that encourages quiet and focus such as asking them to find five insects. You might add that of course they can talk if something important happens, like if they get hurt and need help. Perhaps consider going on a silent walk on your own as well and see how that feels. May a silent walk outdoors with your loved ones offer healing connection and restorative medicine.

Parenting After Loss

Parenting in the midst of and after womb loss can be difficult. We are postpartum, we are grieving, and we are healing from our own trauma. To also tend to the needs of living children can be an added layer to an already overwhelming situation. It is a lot. And if you are having a difficult time, that is understandable. You may be grieving the secondary loss of not being as present a parent as you'd like to be. All you can do—all anyone can do—is the best you can in a given moment. Remember, it is okay to grieve and to show your grief in the presence of living children, as well as grieving with them. It can also be helpful to compartmentalize and make plans to tend to your grief at a certain time and place. Knowing you will tend to your grief at that point may help free you to focus on actively parenting when you need to. Doing so can also help you center yourself and tend to your needs, even in seemingly small ways, at some point in your day. Perhaps engage in self-tending when you first wake up. This can help you feel grounded amidst the demands of parenting. It is a constant and at times tricky and overwhelming dance of self-tending and tending to others who depend on you.

We are part of nature despite how much modern living can leave us feeling disconnected. Being in nature can instantly calm our nervous systems, helping us to feel grounded, centered, and safe. Nature has the power to soften our being, and it has the power to heal our spirits. The following practice is an invitation to connect with Mother Nature and the healing she has to offer you and your loved ones.

GROUNDING RITUAL PRACTICE

A Moment with Nature

For this practice you will need a tree, other plant, or flowers.

The Invitation

Together with your loved ones, plant a tree or remembrance garden in honor of your womb loss. Depending on the outdoor space available to you, you might plant in the ground in your backyard or you might use a planter. Choose a plant that has special meaning to you. If it is a better fit, you might purchase a house plant instead or donate to an organization that will plant a tree on your behalf. If you have the remains from your pregnancy, you might choose to bury them with your plant and find comfort in knowing the life you carried lives on in the life of the plant. You might add other meaningful items in and around the plant, like statues or a wind chime. You might infuse a sense of honoring yourself as well by tying small ribbons to the branches for each loss your body has endured. There is no right or wrong way to do this. Allow your intuition and creativity to guide you, and allow this piece of nature to help soften your grief as it softens your space.

Honoring the Grief of Other Loved Ones

As meaningful as it can be to honor the grief of a partner and living children, so too is honoring the grief of other loved ones who may otherwise feel unseen. This can include your parents, and if you are partnered, their parents, as they grieve what your womb loss means to them. Remember, while you and your loved ones may be grieving the same womb loss, each of you is grieving in your own way and in your own time. Your parents may be grieving the loss of their grandchild or grandchildren, the loss of their role as a grandparent, the plans they may have been making for their time together. They may be grieving your own journey—that you had to endure so much pain—and may be worried for you. It is not your job to take away their grief, their feelings. That is for them to hold and tend to. However, you might consider how you can acknowledge their grief and include them in your family's mourning process, affirming the validity of their grief.

The following practice is an invitation for you and your loved ones to honor your shared experience of womb loss by co-creating a remembrance table—a place to connect to your grief, to your baby/babies, and to one another—much like the altar in the opening story of this chapter. Having a tangible place for your grief can help you feel relief from the weight of carrying it all. It can also help you and your family grieve together, even as you each grieve differently.

GROUNDING RELATIONAL PRACTICE

Co-Creating a Remembrance Table

You will need the following:

- Clean and clear surface (such as a table, countertop, book shelf)
- Cloth for items to rest on (optional)
- Items that are meaningful to you in the context of your womb loss
- Candles or incense (optional)

The Invitation

Together with your loved ones, co-create a remembrance table (also referred to as a memorial table or an altar) that honors your experience of womb loss. You might begin by cleaning the surface of the resting place you have chosen for your items and by playing calming music that connects you to your loss.

Then place the cloth over the surface and take your time adding items that are meaningful to each of you. This may include an urn with your baby's remains, a symbolic urn if you do not have any physical remains, or ultrasound photos and other printed photos. It may include items that convey the love you want to share with your baby, such as clothing or toys that were meant for them. This may include items that honor you and what you have endured, such as a photo of yourself when you were pregnant. If you are part of a faith community, this might include items that are meaningful to that part of your identity. You might include a Jizo statue; though rooted in Buddhist tradition, it is becoming more widely known and beloved by bereaved parents of diverse backgrounds. And you might invite the healing and beautifying power of Mother Nature with items such as flowers or plants, as well as candles and incense. If you have living children, they might choose to add toys that they would have wanted to share with their sibling(s), art they created for their sibling, or other items that feel meaningful to them and their unique relationship to your womb loss.

Once this practice feels complete, you and your loved ones might gather around your remembrance table for a moment of silence, perhaps lighting a candle or incense (if you have living children, you might let them choose an incense stick). Perhaps share a few words about what this remembrance table means to you, recite a prayer, read a poem, or read a book you would have wanted to read to your baby. Then, when you are ready, consider a way to close this practice together. This may be as simple as taking a deep, cleansing breath or blowing out a candle. Please know that a remembrance table and how you interact with it can be dynamic and ever changing. Follow your intuition and honor what feels meaningful.

Offering from the Collective

The following is an offering from a cherished friend who is also my former clinical supervisor. I first met Amanda fresh out of graduate school, and I distinctly remember wishing we were not colleagues so that she could be my therapist. I always looked forward to our supervision sessions, knowing I would be met with her signature warmth and valuable insight. In the many years since, we have supported each other as budding authors, each of us taking our life's passion and channeling it into books meant to nurture softness in a hard world. In thinking of an offering that could tend to you and your loved ones' grief, I knew Amanda would be a valuable resource as a therapist who specializes in both relationships and perinatal mental health.

AN OFFERING BY AMANDA GRIFFITH-ATKINS

Talk Therapy

What it is

Talk therapy (also known as psychotherapy) is a healing modality in which you and a mental health professional, commonly referred to as a therapist or talk therapist, meet on a regular basis to discuss stressors you are experiencing and what shifts might help you improve your mental health or work toward life goals. Generally, the role of a therapist is to hold space for you to feel safe sharing the most vulnerable parts of yourself, offering you their full, undivided attention, compassion, and professional insight. At its essence and ideally, you are able to feel truly seen, heard, and validated and then able to reenter your life feeling capable of addressing the issues that concern you with the emotional support and practical strategies offered in a session. There are many types of therapists who specialize in different clinical areas and approaches, and it may take time to find one who is a good fit for you and your needs. For example, as a marriage and family therapist, I find value in understanding a person from a systemic perspective. English poet John Donne said, "No man is an island," and that perfectly encapsulates what it means to think systemically. Understanding your family, culture, ancestors' journeys, childhood, relationships, and experiences are all key to better understanding who you are in this current moment.

How it can support you

It can be invaluable to connect with a mental health professional in the midst of or in the aftermath of pregnancy and infant loss. They can provide emotional support, resources, and help identify whether you are experiencing any perinatal mood and anxiety disorders (also known as PMADs), which is unfortunately common after birth in general and a heightened risk after pregnancy and infant loss (also known as perinatal loss). Despite perinatal loss being a very common experience, those who experience it often feel reluctant, ashamed, or even scared to talk about it. This sense of isolation can add to already existing challenges of healing from pregnancy and birth, as well as grieving the loss itself. Grief is such a complicated emotion that's often met with clichéd, unhelpful responses (God has a plan, your baby's in a better place now, this just wasn't meant to be, etc.). In your therapist's office, you will be validated, emotionally held, and have the space to openly express all that you're feeling. A therapist will also assess and address any risk for self-harm or maternal suicide, which may include connecting you to a provider who can assess the need for medication as an additional source of support.

If you are partnered, couples therapy can be a helpful resource as you each navigate your own unique process of grieving. In that format, a therapist can help bridge any divides by observing patterns in behavior, communication, or feelings between you and your partner and recommend changes that support the well-being of the relationship. Family therapy can be a chance to explore how the experience of womb loss is impacting other family members, including any living children, who may be grieving both the loss and their role as an older sibling, and parents, who may be grieving their grandchild and their role as grandparents.

A Letter to Our Child

A self-tending practice

When we experience womb loss, we grieve what could have been. Because of this, it's deeply important to honor the way this loss has impacted our lives and the future we envisioned.

If you are partnered, I invite you and your partner to each separately write a letter to your child who has passed. You can include anything in this letter: your emotions, your hopes for their spirit, your commitment to never forget them. Please remember there is no wrong way to do this practice. Co-create the guidelines as needed and give yourself permission to bring to paper what naturally arises within you.

If you feel comfortable, set aside some dedicated time to share your letters with each other. You can read your letter aloud or have your partner read your letter quietly, and vice versa. Honor what feels right for you individually and as a couple. Take some time to reflect on this experience, acknowledging how it feels to speak to your child and share this moment with your partner.

What you do with your letters is up to you, and I encourage you to think about what would feel meaningful. Some bereaved parents I have worked with have found it helpful to bury the letters outside under a beautiful plant or to cut the letters into strips and place them inside a keepsake ornament. Others simply fold the letters and put them in a safe place. Perhaps you'd like to frame the letters and put them on your bedside table or a remembrance table. Or you might decide to do one thing while your partner does something different, which is totally fine. It is important that each of you do what feels most meaningful for yourselves.

If you have living children, and depending on their age, you can invite them to write a letter or draw a picture for their sibling. You and your partner can do this alongside them as a way to honor your loss as a family. Afterward, you can invite them to share what they wrote or drew. You might reflect back to them the thoughts they are sharing, using their words. For example, with a young child you might say, "I see you drew a toy, and I hear you say you would like to share that toy with our baby if you could. That is so thoughtful of you." You can even invite others in your life to write a letter (such as your parents) and expand this practice of tending to hold the larger collective of hearts that are grieving alongside you.

A Gentle Closing

Thank you for being here. For showing up for yourself, your body, and your grief as we explored how our womb loss can also be felt and grieved by those around us. You are not alone in your pain. Even if your loved ones may not know the experience of womb loss with their bodies, their grief is just as valid. May you be gentle with yourself and with them as you all grieve this loss in your own time and in your own ways, honoring what is yours to tend and to hold and honoring what is theirs.

As this chapter comes to a close, I invite you to pause for a few breaths and with the closing verse to help you transition gently back into your life or to the next part of the book. And if anything in this chapter activated a strong response, consider doing something more to feel grounded. This may be an act of self-tending or reaching out to someone you trust for support. Honor what you need in this moment.

I am here, as I am.
And so it is.

You are here.
And we are with you.

CHAPTER 7

Mourning

Do what you need to feel at peace.

I t was like nowhere else I had ever been before, a truly magical place that radiated a sweet kind of sadness interwoven with an essence of serenity and playfulness. Colorful tiny houses at the base of a cement staircase welcomed me and hinted at what was to come. I remember stopping just short of entering this most sacred of spaces. I took in the beauty before me: soft, late afternoon sunlight filtering through the leaves of towering trees, the calming sounds of windchimes singing from the branches, and the fresh, nourishing scent of the native forest.

Taking slow, careful steps, I followed the path that led me farther into Little Spirits Garden. My eyes danced around as I took in all the tiny concrete houses—some painted and decorated with figurines and trinkets, others left bare, though no less moving. Before arriving, I learned that these tiny houses, chosen by the garden's architects as a universal and nondenominational symbol of protection, are offered to families free of charge to support them in grieving and mourning the loss of a pregnancy or an infant. Sprinkled amongst the houses were statues of Jizo (the Buddhist protector of unborn babies and children who die young), fairy doors fastened against tree bases, angel statues, and a stunning sculpture of a pair of hands cradling an infant.

Lorraine Fracy was my guide that day. She is the person who created Little Spirits Garden and also a staff member of Royal Oak Burial Park where it is located. When I first met her in her office, her depth of compassion and genuine warmth moved me to tears. Her essence is reflected in the garden, where she invited me to approach a giant stone sculpture resting underneath a metal pergola. I felt a palpable energy around the stone as I gently glided my hand along the top with intuitive reverence. Lorraine then shared that this beautiful stone is an ossuary, a shared place of rest for cremated remains. She explained that they regularly receive fetal remains from local hospitals, which they cremate in a way that is sensitive to their size and composition. Then, after a simple ceremony of ringing a beautiful, custom-made handbell and sharing some loving words, Lorraine or a coworker opens the ossuary and reverently pours the new ashes in. After learning this, I returned my hand to the stone with a deeper reverence for what it held inside.

Before we left, Lorraine invited me to walk down a path behind the ossuary to an intimate area surrounded by trees. She told me this is where families can release the ashes of their infants if they desire. The energy felt freer here. Wilder. Maybe because it is part of the ancient forest that borders Little Spirits Garden. As we made our way back, we both stopped suddenly. Not more than twenty feet away stood a buck, as still as we were for a moment before continuing on its way. Lorraine and I looked at each other with wide-eyed awe and a shared sense of mystery. As we walked toward the main road, Lorraine told me that in her twenty years working there she had never before seen a deer this far into the park. Once we reached her car, the buck walked out onto the road accompanied by a doe. It seemed as if they, too, knew how special this place is and were drawn to it.

Before leaving, I brought my partner and living children to Little Spirits Garden. We had traveled over 1200 miles to visit, towing our Airstream trailer along the western coast of the United States and then taking the ferry from Port Angeles, Washington, to Vancouver Island in Canada. I felt drawn to visit Little Spirits Garden after reading about it in a 2019 BBC article.[1] I'm so glad I followed that impulse. I watched in awe as my living children bounded through the garden, eager to look at all the houses, especially those with toys inside. That they felt such ease and joy here was a testament to its magical essence. It felt right that they knew this place existed and that our two spirit babies could find a home here too.

~

I left that visit with two cement houses in hand. Lorraine invited me to personalize them and bring both back or just one and keep the other. I have yet to bring myself to unwrap them from their bubble-wrap cocoons. Even though years have passed since my early pregnancy losses, the thought of unwrapping these houses activates some anxiety in me. I feel tightness in my chest. Perhaps it's because unwrapping them would make my losses feel more acute again after the years have softened my memories. I am surprised by my reluctance, *and* I accept that I am not yet ready to mourn in this way. I will continue to wait until it feels right for me. What I know is that my visit to Little Spirits Garden was deeply healing. Seeing all those tiny houses was profoundly affirming. They seemed to say in chorus, with the uplifting spirit of the memorial space: "Your grief is valid. It deserves a special place like this. You are not alone. Look at how many others are grieving with you." And this feels like enough for now.

Mourning Is Showing, Mourning Is Sharing

Whereas grieving is feeling, mourning is showing the grief you feel inside. When you mourn, you allow your grief to manifest outside of you, giving it form and sharing it with the world. Such visible evidence of your grief can help others both know of your loss and that such loss is valid and worthy of mourning. Sharing what you feel inside also helps to lighten the load you carry; you don't have to bear it alone. Whether with Mother Nature, family, friends, acquaintances, or social media, sharing your grief and feeling supported can help soften you, your body, and your emotional pain. The outward expression of the grief we feel inside can be done with others or in peaceful solitude. How might you give outward expression to the grief you feel inside? There is no right or wrong way to mourn, just as there is no right or wrong way to grieve.

If you live in a culture with no strong guidelines for how to mourn pregnancy and infant loss, connect with your body and your intuition and let them guide you. And know that while it is common for rituals to focus on the baby that died, those of us who have experienced womb loss in and with our bodies also deserve to be mourned. The following practice invites you to mourn and release thoughts and feelings you no longer want to carry. May this help create more room for you to breathe and to welcome thoughts and feelings that nourish you.

GROUNDING BREATHING PRACTICE

Breathing into a Stone

For this practice you will need a stone.

The Invitation

In your own time, I invite you to find your way into a comfortable seated position. Please begin as we so often do, by drawing your awareness to your breath, allowing it to follow each inhalation and each exhalation. Allow any other thoughts to melt away. When you feel grounded and centered, I invite you to gently bring the stone to your lips. Inhale through the nose, then let your next exhalation move out through the mouth and into the stone, carrying with it any thoughts, feelings, or felt sensations you no longer want to hold. Inhale through the nose; exhale into the stone. Inhale through the nose; exhale into the stone. You are welcome to continue breathing in this way, allowing each exhalation to carry anything you would like to let go of into the stone. Perhaps consider keeping the rock for a period of time should you want it to hold more for you. Then if it feels right, I invite you to return the stone to the earth. This may be by burying it or throwing it into a body of water. Mother Nature can hold all that you need to release.

Often the most powerful acts are the simplest ones. Know that mourning rituals can be as simple as you would like them to be—even as simple as breathing into a stone. What matters most is what is meaningful to you and the intention you infuse into what you do.

Mourning Baby

If you consider your pregnancy a baby, give yourself permission to honor that to the fullest. Mourning your baby can be instrumental in your grieving and healing process. Simply acknowledging what your womb loss means to you, no matter how short or long your pregnancy lasted, can be powerful medicine. Once you have brought the meaning of your loss into your awareness, you can better decide if and how you might honor it in an external way. Mourning is showing what your baby means to you even if you cannot hold them in your arms. It is maintaining a connection with them that is personal and significant. It is offering them the love you would have given had they lived. There are countless ways to mourn your baby. You can search online with keywords like "memorializing pregnancy loss" or "memorializing infant loss" for ideas. See if anything resonates and trust your own intuition to guide you.

The following practice is an invitation to mourn your baby by choosing an item that will help you maintain a loving connection to them.

GROUNDING MINDFULNESS PRACTICE

A Mourning Ritual for Baby

The Invitation

If and when it feels right for you, choose or create a remembrance item to mourn your baby and place it somewhere you can see each day. This might be an ultrasound photo, a photo of their body, an item of clothing they wore, or even something representative of them like a statue. You can place this item where only you can see it or perhaps where others can too, creating an opportunity for them to ask about your baby. Choosing a remembrance item can make the loss feel more real, and that can be hard. Take your time, and know that you can come back to this practice at a later date if doing it right now feels like too much.

Mourning You

It is essential to mourn ourselves as much as we may mourn the ending of our pregnancies, the loss of our babies. This may seem like a novel idea for those of us who live in societies that focus more on what grows within us, whether a pregnancy ends with living children or loss. If mourning is an outward expression of our grief, what can mourning womb loss look like when we center ourselves? In a form of loss so intimately tied to our own bodies, mourning ourselves can be an act of self-tending and allowing ourselves to be tended to. It can be self-tending, such as self-massage or making yourself a cup of tea. It can be tending from others, such as talking with a therapist, working with a pelvic floor physical therapist, or allowing a friend to pick up your living child from school so you can rest. Such acts honor all that you and your body have endured and continue to endure. Mourning you is, at its essence, honoring your needs. And how different might our experiences be if society acknowledged us and our needs? For example, what if we had pregnancy and postpartum registries instead of baby registries? Or if we had greeting cards acknowledging how hard it can be to get pregnant, to be pregnant, to endure labor, to give birth, to be postpartum, and to be both postpartum and bereaved—not cards only welcoming baby? There is much to unpack here, but for now, consider what it might look like to mourn you, to express any grief for yourself and your experience of womb loss.

But before we can express and share such grief through acts of mourning, we must first acknowledge what our loss means to us and *feel* what our loss means to us. The following is an invitation to connect with and tend to the part of us that carries the grief from our womb loss.

Bearing Witness to You

To bear witness is to hold space for whatever is present with kindness. To offer your full, undivided attention with softness and a willingness to suspend opinions, judgment, and any inclination to "fix." To feel witnessed is to feel safe showing up as you are, sharing what you will, and feeling received. Feeling held.

We can witness others, and others can witness us. Maybe less obvious is that we can also bear witness to ourselves. So, even if you feel alone, know that you can offer yourself the compassionate presence and care you deserve.

The Invitation

When you are ready, arrange two chairs to face each other: one for you to sit in and one left empty. If you prefer to sit on the ground, you can place a pillow or folded blanket in front of you. You might also explore sitting with your back against a wall and see how this feels for your body. If your experience of womb loss was traumatic or if you carry other traumas, having a wall behind you can help to offer a sense of safety in that nothing can surprise you from behind. It may also feel grounding and reassuring to lean back into the wall and feel its solid presence.

Once you feel settled, use your breath or the physical sensation of your body resting on a surface to anchor yourself in the present moment. Then imagine the part of you that gave birth to your loss, to your baby, sitting across from you now. If you have experienced the birth of multiple womb losses, you might choose to connect with all those parts as they sit across from you or invite them to join you one at a time. The invitation here is to sit and bear witness to this most tender part of you. With softness. With kindness. To give this part of you your full loving attention. Perhaps you notice details, like how this part of you looks. Perhaps you gaze into their eyes as you sit in silence. Offer time and space for this part of you to share what they think. What they feel. What they need. And if it feels right, you might begin talking to this part of you. Perhaps telling this part what you would have wanted to hear at that time of the birth. Perhaps sharing how you have been since the birth. Stay with this part of you for as long as it feels right, and when you feel ready to bring this practice to a close, perhaps thank this part of you for enduring the birth, the loss, and making it possible for you to be here in this moment.

Self-Tending Anointing Oil

A Recipe by Eileen S. Rosete and Michelle Goebel-Angel

At the heart of self-tending is reverence for yourself, a deep respect for your entire being—your physical body, emotional body, mind, and spirit—and deep respect for your lived experiences, your resilience, and even your trauma. This recipe was inspired by the work of Felicia Cocotzin Ruiz, curandera and author of *Earth Medicines*, and created to help you know you are worthy of being held in reverence. It is an anointing oil you can use ritually to honor yourself.

Each oil was chosen carefully, with your grief and postpartum healing in mind. Black spruce is a calming needle oil to help you feel rooted, much like the tree it comes from. Rose oil is known to encourage self-love and self-compassion. May it help you honor the courageous softening that grieving and postpartum healing ask of you. Bergamot oil has an uplifting citrus scent to honor your rising after the collapse in grief; it can be part of your process of becoming someone new, someone changed. When using bergamot and other citrus essential oils on the skin, consider covering your skin when outdoors and exposed to sunlight. Finally, jojoba is a slow-growing plant that can live for over a century. May this carrier oil, rich in vitamin E and known to help heal and soften the skin, lend you the wisdom of its years, the healing power of its seeds, and the resilience to reach into your depths.

The power of this recipe is not only in the essential oils but also in the thoughts, energy, and physicality you bring to it. As you touch each object, know this is in honor of you. As you blend the ingredients, know this is in honor of you. And as you use the oils, know this is in honor of you. Infuse this recipe with great love so that it may offer it back to you.

* Jojoba oil
* 6 drops of black spruce essential oil
* 6 drops of rose essential oil
* 6 drops of bergamot essential oil
* Roller bottle (optional)

Before combining the oils, you might pause and anchor yourself in the present moment with a deep breath or by pressing your feet into the earth. Then, with tenderness and at your own pace, add each essential oil to the roller bottle and then fill it with jojoba oil, cap, and label. Gently blend by rolling the bottle between your hands, perhaps closing your eyes and infusing it with intentions for your healing. Alternatively, you can combine the oils in a cup, bowl, or other container around the house. You can also simply add one drop of each essential oil and a few drops of jojoba oil to the palm of your hand.

To use, apply your anointing oil wherever it feels right. You might anoint your lower back to support courage and a sense of feeling grounded. You might anoint your womb space to guide in self-love, self-compassion, and self-tending. And you might anoint your heart to enliven your spirit. As with any oil applied topically, apply a small amount to your skin to gauge any possible reactions. Additionally, you can add drops of your anointing oil to a warm bath or foot bath, soaking for as long as it feels right. And if you feel drawn to use essential oils other than those listed here, allow yourself to honor that urge and make this recipe your own.

Mourning the Future

Just as we may grieve what could have been, so too we can express that grief outwardly and mourn what we had hoped for the future. Consider what you were, and maybe still are, longing for had your pregnancy ended with a living child. This may be the clothes you would have bought, the room you would have decorated, the trips you would have taken. Now, consider how you might express the grief you feel knowing these cannot come to pass. Maybe you will place food on a remembrance table, like the woman in Japan who prepared food her child would have eaten each year had they been alive. Maybe you will choose to celebrate your baby's birthday or estimated delivery date with a cake each year. There is no right or wrong way to mourn. Honor what resonates for you.

The following practice is an invitation to rest. In yoga, Savasana is the final pose at the end of a practice. It is meant to be a pose of rest and an opportunity for your body to integrate all the effort you just made. You, dear reader, have been through so much, and you have come so far. Allow yourself this moment of rest. In a culture that values doing over being, rest is a precious gift to offer yourself. And it is in moments of rest that we may gain clarity for how to mourn in a way that feels true to us.

GROUNDING EMBODIMENT PRACTICE

Restorative Savasana

Restorative poses that include many props for support may take some time to set up. Consider asking a partner or other trusted person to read the following aloud and help with setup if it would feel supportive.

You will need the following:

* Yoga mat
* Bolster
* 2 yoga blocks
* 3–4 blankets

The Invitation

1. Begin by laying down a yoga mat and then a blanket over it to create a soft place to land. Then place a yoga block on its highest height at one end of the blanket and a second block on its lower height in front of the first block. Rest a bolster over the blocks to create a sloped surface for you to lay your back on.

2. When you are ready, come to a seated position on the blanket with your sit bones gently pressed against the bottom edge of the bolster. Take another blanket, fold it in half twice, then roll it on the long edge. Bring the soles of your feet to touch, with your knees pointing to the sides in a butterfly pose, and place the rolled blanket on top of your feet before drawing the sides of the blanket under the legs toward your body for your knees to rest on. Alternatively, you can choose to extend your legs forward and place the rolled blanket under the knees, or bend the knees and place the soles of your feet on the earth.

3. Slowly, lower yourself back onto the bolster and drape a blanket over your body from the neck down to keep yourself warm and help you feel safely cocooned. If it would feel more comfortable, consider adding a pillow under each arm to rest on. You can take one more blanket, folded in half twice, and drape it over your belly to offer this tender part of you extra warmth and a comforting weight.

4. You are welcome to close your eyes or soften your gaze as you allow your body to melt down into the bolster and blankets beneath you. You don't need to do anything except breathe and be. If visually focusing on something helps you feel at ease, perhaps notice the blanket on your belly rising with each inhalation and falling with each exhalation. Allow yourself to feel held as you rest here for as long as it feels right.

5. When you are ready to bring this practice to a close, perhaps take a few deep cleansing breaths before turning to your side and using your arms to gently press yourself up into a seated position.

Mourning Alone

Just as self-tending is as important as being tended to by others, mourning alone is as essential as mourning with others. We can feel especially vulnerable when we are grieving and postpartum. Both are tender times on their own, and are more so when they are experienced together. This can make it easy to feel overwhelmed when you are around other people, especially crowds or amidst fast-paced energy. Consider offering yourself moments of solitude in peaceful spaces to simply be with yourself and to honor your needs without any pressure or distraction from external stimuli. Perhaps notice how expressing your grief alone compares to doing so with others.

The following solo practice is an invitation to turn to the healing power of water. Water is often regarded as a symbol of life, as all living things need water to survive. Water is also a powerful symbol of cleansing and can help you release all that you no longer want to hold.

Water for Releasing

For this practice you will need flower petals.

The Invitation

Connect with water by going to the beach or a local river or stream. If none of these are accessible, you might simply fill a bowl or bathtub with water. When you are ready, I invite you to release the flowers into the water, one petal at a time, allowing each petal to carry with it a thought or a feeling related to your womb loss. You might take a moment to inhale the flower's fragrance before releasing each petal. Watch as the water takes it from you and carries it away. If you are using a bowl or a bathtub, add all the flower petals you feel called to add before removing them and pouring the water out (on plants that could use the water if you have them) or draining the tub. You might find a place outdoors and return the flower petals to nature.

Mourning Together

A supportive community's presence and care are essential to all postpartum healing traditions. The same can be said for postpartum healing after womb loss—maybe even more so given the grief that is present. Mourning with others, especially mourning with others who have experienced womb loss with their bodies, can be profoundly comforting and validating. Mourning in community can look many ways. What is important is the intention of honoring your shared loss and feeling the collective energy of grief and love together. Mourning in community can look like a walk/run event in honor of pregnancy and infant loss, sharing a meal, doing yoga, or taking a drive to the ocean. Mourning with others simply means feeling your grief in the presence of others and expressing your grief together.

The following practice is an invitation to express your grief through a mourning ritual with your loved ones.

A Shared Piece of Art

For this practice, you will need paper and art supplies.

The Invitation

Together with your loved ones—be it a partner, living children, parents, or others—take a moment to slow down and create a piece of art together that honors your shared grief. If you have living children, you might ask them to show you what their grief feels like. Perhaps play soothing music or allow this practice to unfold in silence with space for conversation to arise organically. Before bringing this practice to a close, take some time to look over the artwork together, sharing observations or reflections. Let this be a time for gentle connection and an opportunity for your body and spirit to express themselves.

Offering from the Collective

The following is a heartfelt offering from one of my beloved friends, Katrina, a gifted healer who blends Western psychology with ancient healing traditions. She and I have traveled our womb loss journeys side by side, with Katrina often reminding me of the medicine to be found in the natural world, including the healing power of plants. As she explained to me, it is important to have a reciprocal relationship with plant medicine, to give as much as you take, offering something in return for the healing power plants share. Ritual is one way to do this as you handle plants with reverence and offer gratitude for the support they provide. I invited Katrina, someone well-versed in ritual, to share her lived wisdom here, with the hope that ritual will feel accessible and supportive to you.

Ritual

What it is

A ritual is a practice used to commemorate a significant event. Rituals have been used by human beings in all traditions and cultures since time immemorial to honor beginnings, endings, and the meaningful periods in between. They may be celebratory and joyful or quiet, somber occasions. Some rituals are times to hold space for a range of emotions, including relief, calm, anger, and uncertainty.

How it can support you

Rituals help give form to feelings. They are tangible ways to express and move through the many shifts and challenges we may experience as womb loss survivors. As humans, we animate the physical plane, but loss can also be felt deeply in the mental, emotional, and even spiritual body. Rituals can help us process what is not obvious in the material space by granting tactility to the impalpable.

Flower Ritual for the Womb

A self-tending practice

The intention with this ritual is to honor your womb space, all that it has given and endured. If you do not have a physical womb, know that you still have an energetic womb space, and it and you deserve to be honored.

1. Gather or buy yourself flowers that you love or that are meaningful to you. Place them in water in a space where you will see them for one to three days (more or less depending on how long they last). The flowers should be fresh but not wilting and beyond the budding phase when you use them for the final steps.

2. Each day that you see your flowers—perhaps on your altar, bedside stand, or kitchen or dining table—think of your womb journey.

Give yourself time and space to allow any emotions to rise. Come back to focusing on the beauty of your flowers. In all traditions and cultures, flowers are associated with feminine energy. They are also the reproductive parts of plants. Hence, they are the perfect representation of your own womb space, even if it doesn't always feel that way.

3. Sit or lie down comfortably with your flowers in hand in a space that feels safe to you, preferably outside but maybe an inside space dear to you. You may wish to have other meaningful or comforting things around you—pictures, cozy blankets, or even people or pets (who can hold quiet space and not be distracting) are welcome.

4. Close your eyes. Place or hold the flowers on your body. You may choose to have them touching your womb or your heart space. Notice the sensations, the softness of the petals, and smell of the blooms.

5. Imagine that anything you are ready to let go of from your womb journey is being transferred from your body to the flowers. This may be visualized as a color or felt as a sensation, as perhaps memories of pain, grief, elation, and longing are poured from you into your flowers. Breathe deeply. Take the time you need for this to feel complete.

6. When you are ready, you can say: *I thank you, womb, for creating and holding all that you have held and created.* If it applies, you may also say: *I thank you, womb, for releasing all that you have released. Thank you for your strength. Thank you for your resilience.* Add any other words of gratitude that feel resonant. Then say: *Thank you, Flowers* (you may also say the specific name of the flower or flowers) *for reminding me of the beauty I hold and carry within. Thank you for reminding me of my strength. Thank you for reminding me of my resilience.* Again, add any other words of gratitude that feel resonant. *Thank you for helping me to release what needs to be released from my womb space.*

7. Release the flowers, a symbolic representation of what you would like to let go of from your womb journey, back to the earth by burying them, scattering them, or releasing them to a body of water in nature. In ancient traditions and cultures, earth and water represent the Great Mother.

Hence, we return all that we receive and are ready to let go of with gratitude, as an offering, to She who has given, held, carried, released, and endured all.

As with all rituals, be gentle with yourself throughout the process—before, during, and after. Things you didn't expect may come up to be remembered or released. You may find that—not unlike after other big events, jobs, or projects—you yearn for extra rest, water, or nourishing foods. Do your best to recognize what arises as part of your journey, and honor your needs. This, and any other ritual you choose to do, may take time to feel effective. You may repeat and return to a ritual whenever you need or desire.

A Gentle Closing

Thank you for being here. For showing up for yourself, your body, and your grief as we explored mourning in the context of womb loss—how we can lighten the weight of our grief by showing it and sharing it. Remember that even the simplest and shortest expressions of our grief can be meaningful. And what is meaningful can be healing. May you be gentle with yourself as you explore how to express your grief, how to mourn, in ways that feel safe and comforting to you, doing what you need to feel at peace.

As this chapter comes to a close, I invite you to pause for a few breaths and with the closing verse to help you transition gently back into your life or to the next part of the book. And if anything in this chapter activated a strong response, consider doing something more to feel grounded. This may be an act of self-tending or reaching out to someone you trust for support. Honor what you need in this moment.

I am here, as I am.
And so it is.

You are here.
And we are with you.

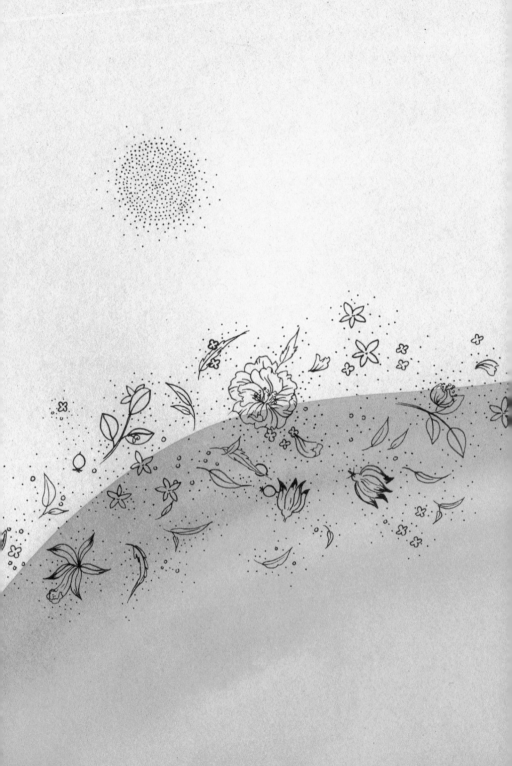

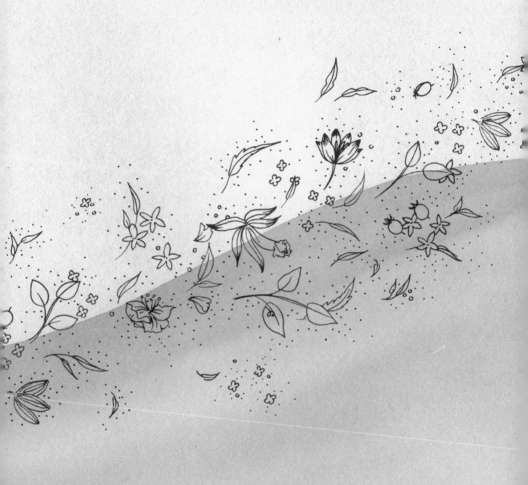

part three
our healing

CHAPTER 8

Postpartum Care After Womb Loss

You deserve to feel cherished.

I first met Aditi on a hot, sunny afternoon at Nose Creek Park in Airdrie, a city just north of Calgary in Alberta, Canada. We were at the second annual Legacy Run/Walk organized by the charitable organization Pregnancy and Infant Loss Support Centre (PILSC), which Aditi had founded. Toward the end of the event, I felt an urge to introduce myself. Honoring my intuition, I approached Aditi, whose story of womb loss and how she was cared for deeply moved me. I share it with you here in the hopes that it will help you know what is possible for your healing process. And so that the world may know what we who endure pregnancy and infant loss are deserving of.

Aditi was pregnant for the second time and facing womb loss for the second time. But unlike her experience of ectopic pregnancy, which was quite sudden and ended with a traumatic hospital experience, Aditi waited five weeks for her body to release this pregnancy at home without intervention. Her mother traveled to be with her during those long weeks. She, too, had experienced womb loss and had experienced it twice. But she did not have support after either loss and wanted to offer that to her daughter. When the time came for Aditi to go into labor, her mother was there, by her side. Ever watchful. Ever sensing her daughter's needs. And when Aditi finally gave birth, her mother held her as they both cried. Aditi could not bring herself to look into the toilet to see what had come forth from her body, but her mother did. And in doing so, the depth of her daughter's pain felt even more real to her.

In time, Aditi made her way slowly to the couch to rest, and her mother sat by her with a jar of coconut oil. "You are postpartum," she told Aditi. "You need to rest and let me take care of you." Her hands followed her words, gently massaging Aditi's exhausted body with long, soothing strokes. What followed for Aditi were weeks of her mother's careful tending with nourishing Indian food, healing touch, and regular reminders for Aditi to rest and take care with her body. This also entailed relinquishing daily household tasks to her mother so that Aditi could rest and grieve.

~

Survivors of womb loss are not commonly identified as postpartum. I came to the realization myself only after experiencing my pregnancy losses. In 2018, I began hosting Our Womb Loss dining events to help others realize that they, too, are postpartum and deserve the same care all who experience pregnancy need after giving birth, including rest, healing touch, warm and nourishing food, and compassionate connection with others. That Aditi's mother knew this and committed herself to Aditi's care, integrating Indian postpartum traditions and helping her name that she was postpartum, was deeply moving. If only the fact that we are postpartum after pregnancy and infant loss were more widely known, how different our world would look. People would better understand how to support us, and we would better understand how to support ourselves.

We, too, are postpartum after pregnancy and infant loss, dear reader. And we are worthy of the same care that all who give birth deserve and need to heal. Know this and let it help guide you in your process of grieving and healing.

Honoring the Postpartum Time

For many, especially those of us in countries like the US where the postpartum time is not yet regarded as a critical period of healing that requires support, there is no clear road map for postpartum healing and absolutely no road map for postpartum healing after womb loss. Nor are there clear cultural guidelines for how to support those of us who endure such loss. It is not something taught in school, even to those whose professions are dedicated to supporting pregnancy and birth, and we may not see it modeled for us in our communities since most suffer this loss alone and in private. But just because such guidance is missing doesn't mean it is not needed. We absolutely need postpartum healing practices that are sensitive to our grief and our trauma. And as much as we can offer such care to ourselves, we also need society to better understand our needs and make tangible efforts to tend to them with us.

The following practice is an invitation to connect with your breath and allow it to help you soften. While simple, this may not be easy, especially if your body carries impressions from experiences that felt traumatic and is ever ready to protect you. Asking it to soften is asking it to be vulnerable, and that can be a big ask. May this practice help you soften in a gradual, gentle way that feels doable. You deserve to feel at ease, even if just for a moment.

GROUNDING BREATHING PRACTICE

Softening Breaths

Grieving, postpartum healing, and healing from trauma cannot be rushed. They are tender processes that need time, space, and support. And you, dear reader, are deserving of all these things and more. Allowing yourself to soften is one way to tend to all three of these processes.

The Invitation

Take your time and find your way into a comfortable resting position, either seated or lying down. Allow your awareness to connect with your breath as it is, your body breathing naturally. There is no pressure to change it in any way. When you are ready, inhale, and as you exhale, think of the word *soften*. Do this three more times if that feels okay for your body, simply noticing what unfolds without actively trying to do anything more.

Inhale. *Soften.*
Inhale. *Soften.*
Inhale. *Soften.*

If you feel pulled to continue this breathing practice, please honor that urge. When you are ready to bring this practice to a close, take a deep breath and press into the parts of you that are touching the ground to help return you to the present moment.

Honoring *Your* Postpartum Time

While the postpartum period is generally defined as the first six weeks after giving birth, since this is about how long it takes for the body to return to a nonpregnant state, it can actually last longer. For some, healing may take months; for others, it may take years. How long it takes your body to heal and return to a nonpregnant state physically and how long it takes to feel like you've returned to yourself mentally, emotionally, and spiritually are unique to you. It took several months for me to feel like myself again after experiencing early pregnancy loss and a solid two years after birth from a full-term pregnancy. During that time, I felt like I was in a fog, present but not quite in my full essence. You might ask those around you who have been pregnant how long they felt their postpartum period lasted to learn the diverse range in experiences. In truth, when you have been pregnant and given birth once, your body cannot fully return to how it was before. Essentially, you are forever postpartum as your body will always be in an "after birth" state. Remember, too, that you are not only postpartum but also bereaved, grieving your womb loss and all the secondary losses related to it. And you may be healing from a loss that felt traumatic. Honoring that we each experience the postpartum time differently and that the postpartum time after womb loss is especially layered and complex can help us tend to our needs with less pressure and more softness.

The following practice is an invitation to bring gentle, compassionate attention to your womb with the intention of supporting its healing process. It was inspired by Tami Lynn Kent, author of *Wild Feminine*, who helped me energetically tend to my womb space after my fifth pregnancy. The soothing sound of her voice over the phone and her kind, intentional presence left a deep impression. I highly recommend her work if you want to explore the pelvic bowl's physical, energetic, and spiritual aspects.

Internal Womb Meditation

As you notice any felt sensations in this practice, remember you can take breaks or choose to stop. It is your choice. Please honor what you need in this moment. And if you no longer have a physical uterus, you are still welcome to engage in this visualization, imagining the energetic presence of your womb within you.

The Invitation

You might begin by playing calming music if that feels supportive to you. Then, taking your time, find your way into a comfortable position, either seated or lying down. Perhaps drape a blanket over your body to offer warmth and a felt sensation of being gently cocooned. When you are ready, bring your awareness to your breath, letting all other thoughts melt away. Perhaps close your eyes or soften your gaze. Then, begin to draw your awareness slowly and gently down your front body to your womb. Sensing into this place, imagine you are standing within your womb and start exploring this space with your senses. What do you notice? Are there any stories or experiences that linger here? Are there any physical aspects such as scar tissue, fibroids, or polyps? If you feel okay staying here a little longer, begin tending to the inside of your womb. Perhaps remove anything that no longer needs to be there and use warm water to gently wipe down all the sides. Perhaps light incense or a plant medicine to support the energetic cleansing of this most sacred of spaces. Then, if it feels right, bring in items that feel comforting, nourishing, and honoring. Maybe plants to soften the space with Mother Earth's healing presence, flowers to adorn your womb in beauty, or a candle to offer gentle warmth and soft lighting. You might even place your hands against the sides of your womb and ask, "What do you need in this moment?" See what emerges. And consider if there is anything you want to say to your womb. Perhaps allow for a conversation to unfold. When you feel ready to bring this meditation to a close, I invite you to offer kind words of acknowledgment to your womb before you deepen your breath and slowly open your eyes if they are closed.

Using Postpartum Resources with Care

Since you, too, have given birth and are postpartum, you can utilize the growing body of resources for postpartum care. There is a beautiful movement unfolding at the moment as many are remembering and sharing long-standing postpartum traditions that have served humankind throughout time, and they apply to you too. However, it is essential to keep in mind that most postpartum resources assume you are postpartum with a living child. As such, they will likely embody a celebratory tone, make countless references to babies, consider a living baby's needs, and include photos of living babies, all of which may activate your grief. So, while there is much to be gained from such postpartum offerings, be aware that they may not be sensitive to those of us who are postpartum and bereaved. Knowing this may help you navigate these resources with the capacity to keep what serves you and leave the rest. If you contact healing practitioners for postpartum care, you might let them know in advance that you are postpartum after loss (simply and with no need to share more details if you don't want to or disclose more information if you feel called to). This can help them tailor their offerings to be grief-sensitive and also trauma-sensitive. You, too, are postpartum, dear reader, and you can keep this truth in mind to guide you in your healing process. You will find a curated list of postpartum books in this book's resources section.

As you tend to your unique postpartum needs, it can be helpful to explore the stories you carry about what pregnancy and birth "should" look like and what you wanted them to look like. Acknowledging the stories we carry and the meanings they embody can help ease our grief and create space for us to receive care during our unique postpartum periods more readily. The following is an invitation to reflect on your reproductive story with compassion.

Your Reproductive Story

It can be hard when there is a disconnect between what we expected to happen and what actually happens. Reflecting on and naming such dissonance in our lived experience can help. To name something that feels hard allows it to soften. May the following help soften the raw edges of your pain as you grieve and as you heal. You will need paper or a journal, something to write with, and art supplies (optional).

The Invitation

We all carry stories of who we are and how we imagined our lives unfolding. Your reproductive story is typically defined as your "narrative of parenthood" and includes your "ideas, hopes, expectations, and dreams about having children and becoming parents."[1] Consider your reproductive story more expansively with the prompts below, and do so with gentleness and kindness for all you and your body have endured. Recognizing your reproductive story and bringing it forth in a tangible way through writing can help you process how womb loss has interrupted it, and it can illuminate why you feel the way you do in the present moment. You are welcome to respond to the prompts with words and images. You might reflect on all, a few, or just one. You might take breaks in between if you feel your trauma being activated. Please honor what you need in this moment.

* Growing up, my family/friends/school/faith/media/culture taught me that my body and my reproductive health . . .

* When I considered being a parent, I imagined . . .

* When I thought about the process of conceiving, I imagined . . .

* When I thought about pregnancy, I imagined . . .

* When I thought about labor and birth, I imagined . . .

* When I thought about the time after birth, I imagined . . .

* When I thought about the end of my fertility, I imagined . . .

Ayurvedic Stuffed Dates

A Recipe by Jenna Furnari

This delicious and nutrient-rich recipe comes from my beloved friend and trusted postpartum doula, Jenna Furnari, who supported me after my fourth pregnancy—one living child and two pregnancy losses later. I hadn't known about postpartum doulas until then. The thought of having someone solely focused on me and my needs sounded divine, especially since fear and anxiety had been constant companions throughout this pregnancy, as I knew the risks and uncertainty involved.

The morning after giving birth to my second living child, I awoke to hear Jenna's sweet voice and the sounds of her cooking through the bedroom door. Though I was still in a haze, I instantly felt held, knowing she was there to prepare nourishing food for my once again acutely postpartum body. I soon heard the door open softly and opened my eyes to see Jenna's warm smile as she placed a small plate of Ayurvedic stuffed dates beside me. I took my first bite and sighed at the warmth, sweetness, and loving intention from Jenna that flowed into me. I felt like I was being honored after all my effort and struggle. And as I teared up, I knew that all who give birth deserve to feel this way.

~

A rich source of fiber, iron, B vitamins, and antioxidants, this simple recipe is a perfect support for postpartum healing and a delectable and nourishing snack throughout the day. This Ayurvedic treat is used to rejuvenate: honey and ghee promote health and strength. Dates nourish healing muscles and are traditionally used to tone reproductive tissues. Whether preparing this for yourself or a grieving loved one, allow your loving intention to flow from you into the food.

- 10 Medjool dates
- 2 tablespoons sunflower butter
- 1 1/2 teaspoons raw honey
- 1 teaspoon ghee or coconut oil

- 2 drops vanilla
- Pinch of mineral salt
- Shredded coconut

Slice the dates down the middle and remove seeds. Set the dates aside. Add sunflower butter, honey, ghee, vanilla, and salt to a small pot and place on the stove over low heat. Heat and stir gently until combined (about 1 minute). Spoon into dates and top with shredded coconut. Serve warm or refrigerate and serve cold. You can make extra and store sealed in the fridge for 2 to 3 days.

Our Shared Postpartum Traditions

We can turn to rich, long-standing postpartum traditions worldwide for guidance and support during our bereaved postpartum healing period. Though they originate from different places, these traditions share an emphasis on the following aspects of postpartum healing: rest, nourishing food and drink, warmth, healing touch, supportive community, and nature—all of which support the body, mind, and spirit as we heal and return to a nonpregnant state. In womb loss, postpartum healing requires all this and an added sensitivity to our loss, our grief, and our trauma. Consider what postpartum healing traditions exist from your own culture or ethnic background that may feel comforting for you. Or perhaps learn about postpartum traditions from other cultures and see if any aspects may feel right for your healing process. You might even research if and what traditions exist for honoring womb loss specifically.

Additionally, consider what self-tending practices exist in your culture and others. These may not necessarily be specific to postpartum care but are nevertheless effective in supporting your healing. For example, one of my favorite forms of tending is going to a local Korean spa and getting a scrub/massage service. Having all the dead skin sloughed off my body and feeling my skin so soft afterward helps me feel renewed, or as one friend said "reborn." Also, being in community with so many other female bodies affirms that our bodies are all quite similar and what may not be considered "ideal" is, in fact, the norm.

All that said, start with tending to your basic needs, including hydration, nourishing food, rest, and sleep. Perhaps set up bottles of water by your bedside the night before so you are ready to hydrate the next day and have nutrient-dense, no-prep snacks like nuts at the ready. Perhaps have a food train or food delivery service take care of your meals so that you can focus on resting and sleeping. The following practice is an invitation to allow yourself to be guided in resting deeply.

GROUNDING EMBODIMENT PRACTICE

Guided Full Body Relaxation

Savasana, the final resting pose in yoga, can be an incredibly vulnerable state: you are lying down, chest open, arms at your sides, legs stretched out, and usually the eyes are closed. For trauma survivors, hypervigilance (constantly scanning for danger) is a normal state of being, so resting in a pose as vulnerable as Savasana requires courage and a great deal of trust to feel safe enough to rest. If your experience of pregnancy loss feels traumatic, remember that you are in full control of this practice and can make any adjustments you need to feel safe. If it feels hard to be in your body right now, the site of this most intimate of losses, that is completely understandable. Anchor yourself in the present with your breath, and see if this guided meditation can offer you some solace from your pain. If at any point you feel your trauma is being activated, consider deepening your breath or pressing down into the earth to signal to your body that you are, in fact, safe. You can also choose to stop completely. Please honor what you need.

You will need the following:

- Yoga mat
- 1–2 blankets
- Bolster or another blanket
- Pillow or additional blanket
- Eye pillow (optional)

The Invitation

Given the guided nature of this meditation, you might ask a loved one to read the directions aloud to you, or if you are alone, you can record yourself reading the directions and then play it back. In a space that ideally is quiet and free of interruption, lay your yoga mat down and place a blanket on top of it to create a soft place for you to land (if you do not have a yoga mat, you can lie on a blanket, sofa, or bed). Then, taking your time, find a comfortable position lying on your back, with your head resting on a pillow or a folded blanket. You might place a bolster or rolled blanket under your knees if you have back pain and a blanket over your body to help you feel warm and safely cocooned. You might also place an eye pillow over your eyes or forehead. If this is uncomfortable, you can find another resting position, perhaps sitting on a folded blanket with your back to a wall. Then, when you are ready, close your eyes or soften your gaze. There is nowhere else you need to be other than here, now, breathing.

When you are ready, take a few deep breaths. Notice the parts of your body that are touching the surface below you. Know that resting and allowing yourself to be held by the earth below is okay. When it feels right, bring your awareness to your scalp. Soften this area, imagining every strand of hair resting easily against your head. You might stay here for a few breaths before allowing your attention to move slowly down to your forehead and allowing this area to soften. Let any lines of worry or concern melt away. And breathe.

Slowly allow your awareness to flow down to your eyelids and eyes, allowing these parts of you to soften. Allow your eyes to rest. They don't need to do anything right now. Next, invite your awareness to your jaw, allowing it to soften as you let your tongue relax down from the roof of your mouth. You might even open your mouth and move your upper and lower jaws in opposite directions to help loosen any tension you are carrying there.

Taking your time, allow your awareness to flow down into your neck, shoulders, and back, letting these parts of you feel heavy and sink into the earth—first your upper back, then your middle back, and your lower back. Imagine any tension or pain you may be carrying here melting out of your body and into the ground below, knowing that Mother Earth can hold anything and everything that no longer serves you.

When you are ready, slowly draw your awareness into both arms, hands, and all your fingers. Let these parts of you feel heavy and sink into the earth. They don't need to do anything right now. Allow them to rest.

Then, draw your awareness back up your arms and into your chest and heart center. Breathe and allow these areas to soften. It is said that grief is stored here and that intense grief can even shift the heart's muscles. See if you can allow any stress or tension you are holding here to melt down through your back and into the earth, leaving you to feel a little lighter and more at ease. If you birthed your loss recently, your breasts may be engorged and may even be lactating. It may be hard to keep your attention here for these reasons, and that's okay.

At your own pace, draw your awareness to your womb space. Depending on where you are in your journey, it may feel particularly tender and hard to keep your attention here. See if you can take a few more breaths without any pressure to change how you feel. You might notice body memories arise or maybe thoughts or feelings you haven't experienced in a while. If you birthed your loss vaginally, you might notice sensations or memories connected to that part of your body. Whatever comes up, try to notice without judgment or attachment, much like you would observe a leaf flowing past you on a stream or a cloud floating by in the sky. Simply notice and breathe. If strong feelings or sensations are coming up for you, allow your breath to deepen or press down into the earth to help you feel grounded. Remember that you are in full control and can come out of this meditation at any time.

Finally, if it feels right, draw your awareness into your legs, feet, and all your toes. Allow these parts of you to feel heavy, sinking into the earth. They don't need to do anything right now. Let them rest, allowing any tension here to flow down and into the ground, leaving your body feeling lighter. Stay here as long as you need to, allowing your body to rest in Savasana. Allow your body to integrate your thoughts, feelings, and physical experiences while you rest.

When you are ready to bring this practice to a close, you can take a full-body breath, raising both arms up and overhead with your next inhalation as you reach in the opposite direction with your legs, feet, and toes. As you exhale, you can return your arms to your sides and relax your lower limbs. Roll to your side, allowing the bottom arm to rest under your head like a pillow as you take a few breaths. Then, gently press both palms into the earth as you come up to a seated position, slowly opening the eyes if they were closed.

Tending to Our Mental Health

It is essential for those of us who endure womb loss to tend to our mental health and to have the support to do so in order to continue living and live meaningfully. A growing body of research validates what many of us have come to know firsthand: that womb loss at any stage of gestation can affect short- and long-term mental well-being.[2] If left untreated, it can cause significant distress not only for us but also for our families and even lead to death.[3] As was mentioned in chapter 3, perinatal mood and anxiety disorders (PMADs) is an umbrella term for serious mental health conditions that make daily functioning difficult and can lead to self-harm. Perinatal mood and anxiety disorders, which impact an estimated one in seven women in the US and are more likely to occur in women of color, can also be experienced by birth partners of any gender, an additional stressor to an already overwhelming situation.[4] There is no single cause for PMADs, which can be attributed to changes in hormones during and after pregnancy, limited or lack of social support, stressful or traumatic life events (including womb loss and race- and gender-based discrimination), a personal or family history of mood or anxiety disorders, and intimate partner violence.

It can be hard to know what a "normal" postpartum experience is and when to reach out for support, especially if you have never been postpartum before and are now both postpartum and bereaved. What follows is a brief overview of PMADs. If you suspect any of these conditions apply to you, whether mild or severe, please know that it is not your fault and that you deserve support. If you are in crisis and have thoughts or intentions of harming yourself or dying by suicide, please put this book down and call your doctor, local emergency number, or national emergency hotline. If you are not in crisis but struggling to function on the most basic level, consider getting care from a trained mental health professional who can offer emotional support, assessments, and any necessary referrals. Except for bipolar mood disorders, which usually require lifelong treatment, PMADs are considered temporary and treatable with such support. Organizations such as Postpartum Support International and Pregnancy and Infant Loss Support Centre offer an abundance of resources on an international scale, including helplines, virtual one-on-one and group support, and provider directories (see the resources section in this book). Also, consider finding a provider who has earned the Perinatal Mental Health Certification (PMH-C) with Postpartum Support International to ensure they are qualified to support you. This includes a spectrum of professionals, from therapists to doulas, nurses, doctors, support group leaders, and peer supporters.

Depression: Depressive symptoms during pregnancy (prenatal depression) or postpartum (postpartum depression) include persistent and intense feelings of sadness, fatigue, anxiety, overwhelm, anger, irritability, emptiness, guilt, worthlessness, loss of interest in things previously enjoyed, crying, eating and sleeping more or less than normal, withdrawing from support networks, and thoughts of self-harm or death by suicide.

Anxiety: Symptoms during pregnancy (perinatal anxiety) or postpartum (postpartum anxiety) include persistent, all-consuming worry that something bad will happen; difficulty resting, sleeping, and eating; racing heart and thoughts; shortness of breath, dizziness, and nausea.

Obsessive-Compulsive Disorder (OCD): Symptoms during pregnancy (perinatal obsessive-compulsive disorder) or postpartum (postpartum obsessive-compulsive disorder) include repeated sudden and intrusive images and thoughts (obsessions) that are scary and usually related to the safety of a living baby, as well as feeling horrified about obsessions and compulsive behavior to reduce obsessions.

Postpartum Post-Traumatic Stress Disorder (PPTSD): Symptoms include flashbacks and intrusive re-experiencing of an event(s) during or after childbirth that was experienced as traumatic; avoiding anything associated with said event(s); persistent irritability; difficulty sleeping; exaggerated startle response or hypervigilance (being constantly alert to potential danger); feeling disconnected; and anxiety or panic attacks.

Bipolar Mood Disorders (Bipolar 1 Disorder and Bipolar 2 Disorder): Symptoms include extreme mood swings involving emotional ups (hypomanic or manic episodes) or downs (depressive episodes) that can last weeks or even months and hinder functioning and relationships. Hypomanic and manic episodes look like high levels of physical and mental energy, with hypomania being a milder form of mania. According to Christine Mark-Griffin, LCSW, PMH-C: "It may be confusing to know if someone is experiencing a bipolar mood disorder because it can feel positive and fun to be around them. For example, during a manic episode, someone may experience feeling very happy or elated, talking very quickly, feeling full of energy, feeling self-important, feeling full of great ideas, and having important plans. They may also be easily distracted, irritated, or agitated."[5] Many women are diagnosed with bipolar depression and/or mania for the first time during or after pregnancy.

Postpartum Psychosis (PPP): Symptoms include thoughts or beliefs that are not true (delusions); seeing images, hearing voices, or smelling things that are not present (hallucinations); confusion; paranoia; and hyperactivity. While regarded as temporary and treatable with professional support, this is a severe mental illness that is considered an emergency because the individual may be at risk for harming themselves and others, making immediate assistance imperative.

The following practice is an invitation to find solace in nature and simplify what can feel like an overwhelming time to a single moment with a single task.

GROUNDING RITUAL PRACTICE

A Touch of Nature

Ritual does not always have to be deep and serious. It can spring from spontaneous, carefree acts done with loving intention. May the following support you in enduring the hard moments with love. For yourself. For your grief. For your postpartum body.

The Invitation

Though simple, this practice may not be easy, especially if you feel any of the symptoms just listed. This may require you to reach deep into your resilience. When you are ready, go outside and place your bare feet on the bare earth—whether on dirt, grass, sand, or maybe in a stream, lake, or ocean. Wherever you can find a break from concrete, let the soles of your feet touch the earth, allow Mother Nature to hold you, and simply be. If it is not easy to access a safe, clean part of nature, consider connecting with nature in another way that is doable for you. Find nature within the space you are in—perhaps sitting with a houseplant and touching its leaves or locating other natural materials in your space, like a wood floor or cotton fabric. We are of nature, though we often live disconnected from it. Returning home to Mother Nature can help ease even the most painful moments in ways that escape words. Allow yourself to be held in her embrace in whatever way you can connect with her.

Create a Postpartum Plan

Creating a postpartum plan for womb loss is just as important as creating a birth plan for womb loss. This can be a simple but no less thoughtful document that outlines how you can resource yourself and allow your community to tend to you so you can focus on resting, grieving, and healing. You can search online with keywords like "postpartum plan" for ideas on what to include, but keep in mind that you will likely find information tailored to those who are postpartum with a living child. What follows are some items to consider prioritizing. You can enlist the help of a partner or other support person if you like.

- Childcare if you have living children (including transportation to and from school and activities)

- A meal train, organized by a support person, to last for as long as four to six weeks or more, and/or a subscription to a meal delivery service (including postpartum-specific meal delivery)

- Preparation of bottles of water to ensure adequate hydration each day

- Help with cleaning, laundry, grocery shopping, and other household chores
- Lactation consultant if you are lactating to support you with expressing or suppressing
- Mental health professional to support your mental well-being and monitor for signs of PMADs
- Pelvic floor physical therapist to support the healing of your pelvic floor and diastasis recti

Your Directory of Support

The intention for this practice is to reflect upon and identify the relationships that can support you in this time of need and bring you ease knowing who you can turn to. A directory of support can also make it easier for those around you to assist you in truly helpful ways. This can be a dynamic document you revise and update to reflect your changing needs. You will need paper and something to write with.

The Invitation

Take your time with this practice and ask someone to assist you if that feels supportive. If you are partnered, it can be helpful to do this together. Consider who in your life could help you emotionally and practically during your postpartum period. These can be family members, friends, coworkers, or even hired professionals. Create a list that you and those around you can easily reference when you need support—maybe posting it on your fridge—and include this information:

- Name
- Phone
- Email
- What they can offer (physical, emotional, or practical support like grocery shopping, organizing a meal train, doing laundry, caring for living children, etc.)

Offering from the Collective

The following is an offering from my beloved friend and Ayurvedic postpartum doula Jenna. She was my postpartum doula, and I shared earlier how her kind presence, delicious postpartum food, and loving intention helped me understand what I missed in my previous postpartum periods—what everyone who births deserves. What I didn't share earlier was how the simple act of taking a bite into her Ayurvedic stuffed dates changed my life. In that moment of being so deeply nourished, the seeds for my Our Womb Loss events, this book, and my becoming a postpartum doula were planted. I knew I wanted to help others feel the way Jenna helped me feel that morning: held in love. May her offering here help you know that the ancient healing system of Ayurveda can also support you in your grieving and healing process.

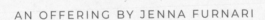

AN OFFERING BY JENNA FURNARI

Ayurvedic Postpartum Care

What it is

Ayurvedic postpartum care is a system of deep, integrated healing that looks at the whole individual and honors forty-two days of rest immediately after giving birth. Ayurveda, which originated in India and is one of the world's oldest medical systems, uses holistic measures that include bodywork, diet, meditation, and gentle yogic practices to bring body-mind balance to someone who is postpartum. After birth, your body goes through tremendous physiological and emotional highs, lows, strain, and stress no matter how long you were pregnant and even when the pregnancy ends in loss. The mission of Ayurvedic care is to restore you so you can function, feeling grounded and well-supported.

How it can support you

Ayurveda uses the system of the three doshas—vata, pitta, and kapha—which looks at each unique individual through the lens of the five universal elements—ether, air, fire, water, and earth. The three doshas influence everything about us, including personality, aging, and digestion. With childbirth, loss, and grief, the body experiences an imbalance of the vata dosha. Ayurvedic care focuses on soothing this dosha, such as with warm, freshly cooked foods that gently build back the body's strength. Thorough digestion can then begin to take place on both physical and emotional levels. Similarly, a simple routine, rest, receiving bodywork, and full emotional support also help you to navigate the trials of grief during the postpartum time. All of these are at the heart of Ayurveda's support for birth and loss.

Abhyanga Self-Massage

A self-tending practice

Abhyanga massage is a cornerstone of Ayurvedic postpartum care and can be used by anyone. This ritual provides several benefits, including a reduction in stress and anxiety and deep healing across all levels of the body. All that is needed is quality sesame or almond massage oil (those two are my favorite for this). These oils are warming and grounding, qualities those who are grieving and postpartum need. Given all the oil you can use, I recommend doing this self-massage in the bathroom.

* Perhaps close the door to the bathroom to help keep it warm, light a candle, and turn on some soft, calming music.

* Take a warm shower or bath while the bottle of oil warms in a sink or pot of hot water.

* After a 10- to 15-minute soak in the tub, you can dry off and sit on a towel on the floor.

* Spend 10 to 20 minutes massaging an abundant amount of the warm oil onto your body using long strokes with moderate pressure. You can start with the soles of the feet and make your way up the legs, hips, and buttocks.

- If you feel comfortable applying touch to your womb space, you can use the oil to gently massage this part of you clockwise.

- Then, you can use long strokes from your hands up your arms and into your armpits.

- Finish with long strokes from your head and face to your heart.

- This can be followed by dressing in enough layers to keep the body warm and comfortable while the healing oils soak into your body.

A Gentle Closing

Thank you for being here. For showing up for yourself, your body, and your grief as we explored long-term postpartum care after womb loss. Given the lack of clear and strong cultural guidelines for how to cope with womb loss, it can be helpful to remember that you are postpartum and deserve the same things all who give birth need to recover from conceiving, gestating, laboring, and birthing. *And*, remember that your postpartum body is also grieving. May you be gentle with yourself as you tend to your postbirth, postloss body and as you honor your postbirth, postloss needs in the weeks, months, and years ahead. You deserve to feel cherished.

As this chapter comes to a close, I invite you to pause for a few breaths and with the closing verse to help you transition gently back into your life or to the next part of the book. And if anything in this chapter activated a strong response, consider doing something more to feel grounded. This may be an act of self-tending or reaching out to someone you trust for support. Honor what you need in this moment.

I am here, as I am.
And so it is.

You are here.
And we are with you.

CHAPTER 9

How to Support Survivors

Community is essential.

T
here were five of us in the car that beautiful, sunny day in Mountain View, California—five bereaved mothers chatting and laughing in a zippy blue Tesla. The energy in the car was lighthearted, following a hike, a tea ceremony, and forest bathing in the stunning Rancho San Antonio Open Space Preserve. Most of us had attended a pregnancy and infant loss retreat four months prior, and this gathering emerged from a longing to feel that sense of community again.

Earlier that morning, we were joined by a sixth bereaved mother. We felt solace being together despite our experiencing womb loss in different ways at different times. Some of us were years out from our loss, while others had given birth recently. One in our group was fourteen months postpartum after birthing her third living child; another, who had birthed her stillborn son shortly before his due date, was pregnant again and unexpectedly so. One was grieving the end of her attempts to conceive and carry a pregnancy, and another was considering which fertility treatment would be the right next step for her. One was grappling with the end of her relationship with her partner, while another was present to finally connect with the memory of her daughter, who died many years earlier after medical complications in her third trimester.

Despite our differences, our shared grief softened any boundaries between us. Being together made our pain feel a little more bearable, and it was healing to be on the ancestral homeland of the Muwekma Ohlone Tribe, taking in the crisp winter air, open fields of green grass, rolling hills, and ancient trees, all against the backdrop of soft white clouds in a bright blue sky. It was soothing to the soul to walk, drink warm tea, mindfully eat nourishing chocolate bars, feel the dirt with our bare feet, and close our eyes as we sat amongst the trees.

After our time in nature, we decided to brunch at a local farmers market. This is how five of us ended up in the zippy blue Tesla. During the drive, one friend began talking about her most recent of nine first-trimester pregnancy losses. She asked the group if we'd like to see a photo of her baby. I turned from the front passenger seat to the sounds of oohing and ahhing. We each took a moment to look at the picture on our friend's phone as she looked on with an expression of profound tenderness, no different from a parent looking at a photo of their living child. The photo showed her baby's little body shortly after it had left hers—her baby's existence confirmed and forever preserved in that image.

~

Sharing such pictures can feel awkward, uncomfortable, or even scary because you may not know how the images will be received. That our friend felt safe enough to share such a precious photo with us was an honor. That we could receive her baby's photo with warmth and enthusiasm *and* hold space for her deep grief at the same time showed me the healing power of community. It showed what is possible for our world. And I hope sharing the memory of this moment can help you know what is possible for you too.

Grieving and postpartum healing after the trauma of womb loss are processes that unfold with no set progression, clear timeline, or definitive end. And that can feel daunting. Scary. Overwhelming. But as our time together that day reminded me, we are not alone as we grieve at our own pace and heal in our own way. In your process of becoming—someone different, someone changed—after experiencing a loss as impactful and traumatic as ours, know that it is essential to feel held in community. To see your pain reflected in the eyes of others who *know*. To feel safe talking about your loss and your grief, trusting you will be received with compassion. To hear words of comfort and embodied understanding. When our womb loss unmoors us, a safe and supportive community reassures us that we can find our footing again. In our own time and our own way. But never alone.

Simple Connection

The simplest acts can often be the most meaningful and memorable. When it comes to self-tending and tending to other womb loss survivors, let it be simple. Let it be sincere. And let it be gentle.

- Simple and specific words of comfort, such as "How are you doing right now?" or "How are you feeling today?" can feel less overwhelming than asking a more general "How are you?"

- Simple acts with consent, like offering and giving a hug, can convey more than words.

- Simply being present can allow space for all that is hard to explain to exist in the silence. And it's okay to name your uncertainty while affirming your caring intention: "I'm not sure what to say or do to help, but I am here for you."

The following is an invitation to practice simplifying by focusing on your breath as you engage in gentle movement.

GROUNDING BREATHING PRACTICE

Breathing with Gentle Stretching

The Invitation

When you are ready, find a comfortable position seated on the earth or at the edge of a chair with your feet flat on the ground. Inhale, and as you exhale, lower your head gently down toward your right shoulder. Inhale as you raise your head to center, and exhale as you gently lower your head toward your left shoulder. Inhale and raise your head back to center. Continue breathing with this simple movement for as long as it feels right. You might also let your head rest to the side for a few breaths, allowing each exhale to deepen the stretch and relieve tension. Listen to and honor your body's needs. To bring this practice to a close, return your head to center, bring the palms of your hands to rest over your heart if that feels resonant, and take a deep cleansing breath.

Reverence

Reverence, which means "a feeling of deep respect or admiration for someone or something," is essential to grieving and healing after womb loss.[1] Reverence for your postpartum body, your needs, your grief. Reverence for other womb loss survivors, their postpartum bodies, their needs, and their grief. This is a word you have seen throughout this book. It is a word that needs to be integrated into prenatal and postnatal care the world over, for all who have and will experience womb loss are worthy of dignified care that includes kind eye contact, soft language, gentle touch, and respect for the pain and risks we endure.

The following practice is an invitation to offer reverence to your body, acknowledging all it has been through.

GROUNDING MINDFULNESS PRACTICE

A Blessing for Your Body

Connecting with your body is a process and one that may not be smooth or easy in the midst of or after womb loss. May this practice support you in nurturing a relationship with your body that is both gentle and reverent. You will need paper and something to write with.

The Invitation

Find a quiet place to sit and rest for a moment. Allow your body to settle into the space, perhaps noticing the parts of you touching the ground and feeling the earth's energy rooting you, holding you in the here and now. Then, when you are ready, write a blessing for your body. Allow this blessing to be meaningful, no matter the length or form. It may be as simple as one word. It may be a few lines. You can refer to the Closing Blessing at the end of the book or look to your own life for inspiration. If you are part of a faith or spiritual tradition, you might consider words and phrases from it that resonate here. Once you have written your blessing, I invite you to read it aloud, focusing on each word and its vibration, perhaps placing one or both hands over your heart or womb as you do. You might also record yourself reading your blessing so that you may listen to it with your eyes closed. Your body has been through so much. You have been through so much. Both deserve reverence.

Space

Space is another essential element for healing after womb loss: personal space and communal space. Space to pause, breathe, feel, and think before we make decisions. Space to rest and grieve after we've given birth. Space in society to address the topic of womb loss with compassion and listen to our experiences of it. It is time to create space to reevaluate language about female reproductive health and space in research to address it adequately. And it is time for education systems to create space in their curriculum for quality training to support womb loss survivors. Space is healing, and we need more of it.

The following practice is an invitation to offer yourself more space in your day by making meaningful choices that slow the pace and protect your energy.

GROUNDING REFLECTION PRACTICE

Spaciousness

It can be easier to soften and feel at ease when there is less pressure and more spaciousness in our days. Space to breathe and simply be. Space to connect with our bodies and hear their needs. Space to tend to our grief and our postpartum healing. May the following help you access your agency and make meaningful choices about how your day unfolds. You will need paper and something to write with.

The Invitation

When you are ready, find your way into a comfortable resting position. Perhaps take a moment to ground yourself by pressing down into the parts of you touching the earth. Remind yourself that Mother Earth is ever present and ready to support you. Then, begin to reflect on and write down your schedule for the day. What needs tending? Who needs tending? Write down what comes to mind so your day is laid out clearly in front of you. Now, consider how you might create more spaciousness. Perhaps there are items you can say "no" to, crossing off and releasing commitments or shortening the time you dedicate to them. Perhaps you can delegate to others so you have less on your plate. Perhaps move things around so you have more space between tasks or appointments and can transition slowly between them. It is okay to protect your time and energy. In fact, it is essential to be protective of yourself so that you can have the capacity to tend to your own needs. Your time and energy are precious. When possible, give them only to what is meaningful and deserving.

A Hug in a Bowl: Chickpea Curry

A Recipe by Lucy Kupferstein

In the early days of my loss, my baby, whom we named Sig Hayes, was all I could think about. I found it hard to eat anything, let alone nourish my body. But I knew from my work and personal experience that certain foods could promote my body's natural ability to heal. I wanted what felt like a hug in a bowl, something that would heal my system and my heart. Curry was the first thing that came to mind when I thought of a dish with those elements. This "throw everything in the pot" meal was easy enough to manage on my own, and it carried me through the difficult days of grieving. I hope this recipe can bring the same comfort to you in your time of need, whether you make it yourself or a loved one does so for you. I hope that this dish can also offer comfort to those in your life who know the pain of womb loss as you share the recipe or cook the dish for them.

~

This meal is rich in healing properties, such as its concentration of heart-healthy fats and vegetables. Turmeric contains a powerful active compound called curcumin, which has anti-inflammatory and antioxidant benefits for healing our postpartum wombs. Broccoli and kale are nutrient-dense cruciferous vegetables and great sources of vitamin C, which boosts our body's immune function. Finally, coconut milk is considered a healthy fat containing medium-chain triglycerides, known for their quick absorption into the bloodstream that then turns into energy your body can use, and lauric acid, which has been shown to have positive effects on the heart by reducing blood pressure and oxidative stress.

- 1 tablespoon of coconut oil
- 1 medium yellow onion, diced
- 3 cloves of garlic
- 1 ½ tablespoon of grated fresh ginger (the more ginger you add, the more aromatic)
- 4 tablespoons of red curry paste
- 1 teaspoon of turmeric powder
- 1 ½ teaspoons salt, or more to taste
- 1 sweet potato, peeled and cubed
- 2 cups of broccoli florets
- 1 red bell pepper, seeded and diced
- 1 15-ounce can of chickpeas (garbanzo beans)
- 2 13½-ounce cans of full-fat coconut milk
- Juice of 1 lime
- 2 cups of roughly chopped kale
- ¼ cup of chopped cilantro

Heat the oil in a large pot over medium heat. Add onion and sauté until translucent. Then add the garlic and ginger and cook for 1 more minute. Add the turmeric powder and sauté 1 to 2 minutes more until fragrant.

Add the sweet potato, broccoli, red bell pepper, and chickpeas to the pot. Pour in the coconut milk, red curry paste, and salt, and stir well. Bring to a boil, then simmer for about 10 minutes or until the sweet potatoes are tender.

If you want a thicker consistency, you can whisk together 1 tablespoon of cornstarch with 2 tablespoons of water in a small bowl and stir into the curry.

Lastly, add the squeezed juice of 1 lime and the chopped kale; stir until wilted. Season with more salt if needed. Serve over brown rice and top with freshly chopped cilantro.

Protected Bereavement Leave

The postpartum period after womb loss is a high-needs time, and you are deserving of practical support so that you have space to grieve and time to heal. This includes time off work, though many may not think to stay home, especially after early pregnancy loss. While it is still rare to have paid bereavement leave mandated for reproductive loss, it does exist. The following four countries have bereavement laws specifically for pregnancy loss: New Zealand (three days of paid bereavement leave for losses beginning at conception), the United Kingdom (two weeks of paid bereavement leave for losses at 24+ weeks), India (six weeks of paid leave following the day of a miscarriage), and the Philippines (sixty days paid leave after miscarriage).[2] Such laws offer practical support to survivors by allowing them protected time off without worrying about the financial impact. They also help entire societies acknowledge the profound significance of womb loss and, in turn, reduce social stigma. Healing from womb loss is an essential blend of self-tending and tending from your community. You deserve to tend to your grief and your postpartum body and to have the systemic support to do so. Know that womb loss is a valid reason to take time off work and that some countries and companies already honor this. Consider exploring your options for taking time off, ideally with pay; you might want a support person to help you with this.

In a world that still has a long way to go to offer us systemic support, it is essential we offer ourselves and other womb loss survivors softness and soft places to land. The following practice invites a physical softening of the body. May it offer you a moment of reprieve from all you are carrying.

Resting with Legs on a Chair

The following is a yoga pose I turn to often. As explained by Jane Austin, a certified yoga teacher, trainer, and founder of the prenatal yoga school Mama Tree: "This posture allows the femur bones to drop into the hip sockets and helps release the psoas. This, in turn, initiates the relaxation response in the body."[3] The moment I come into this pose, it's as if my whole body sighs in relief. I hope this can be true for you as well.

You will need the following:

- Chair (or sofa, ottoman, or coffee table)

- 2 blankets

- Eye pillow (optional)

The Invitation

When you are ready, lay a blanket on the ground in front of the chair. Sit on the blanket with the left side of your body against the front edge of the seat. Carefully lower your right side to the ground and slowly roll onto your back as you bring the backs of your legs to rest on the seat. Allow your knees to be at or close to a 90-degree angle. Drape a blanket over your body to create a warm cocoon for yourself, and place the eye pillow over your eyes or forehead. Let your arms rest at your sides, palms up if that feels okay. Allow your body to feel heavy, melting further into the chair and the earth with each exhalation. Rest here as long as it feels right for you. To come out of this pose, slowly roll to one side as you bring your legs off the chair. Rest here for a moment before gently using your hands to press yourself up to a seated position.

The Gift of Solitude

Solitude can be essential to grieving and healing from womb loss. While it is so easy to feel alone in the midst of and after womb loss for many reasons we have already touched on, such as the prevailing stigma that shames and discourages survivors from reaching out for help, choosing to be alone to honor your needs can feel different. This is solitude, an intentional refuge from the pace and pressures of daily life. It is allowing yourself quality space and time to simply be. To hear yourself think and to feel your feelings without concern for others.

Years ago, when I was first beginning to conceptualize my dining events for womb loss, I sat next to a nurse on a flight. As we chatted, I told her about my plans to honor womb loss survivors. She shared that she had experienced an early pregnancy loss many years ago, and the best gift she and her husband received then was a paid hotel stay so they could get away. I remember the emotion with which she shared how meaningful that gift was to her. It allowed her and her husband to heal in solitude together at a time when it was difficult to live day to day.

When it can be so hard to extract ourselves from the typical flow of our daily lives, especially if we have many other responsibilities (living children, elderly parents, jobs, etc.), how might we offer ourselves solitude? How might we help other womb loss survivors access solitude? The following practice is an invitation to channel your grief into a physical item, creating an anchor you can turn to in even the most fleeting moments of solitude—something you can hold and something that lets you feel held in return.

GROUNDING RITUAL PRACTICE

Remembrance Jewelry

Giving a physical form to your grief can help you feel connected to your loss in a way that feels comforting. Having it be in the form of jewelry that can rest on your body can offer a tangible connection that feels both intimate and easy to access when you need something to touch to anchor you. So that you may feel grounded. So that you may feel secure. Even if just for a moment. Know that you have the power to create such meaningful items for your healing.

The Invitation

Remembrance jewelry is, as the name implies, jewelry that helps you remember. Remembrance jewelry for womb loss tends to focus on baby, but the invitation here is to choose or create jewelry that helps you remember your womb loss *and* your resilience—that honors whatever your loss means to you *and* that you endured it or are enduring it still. This can be a necklace, a bracelet, a ring, earrings, or other adornment. You can do an internet search with keywords such as "remembrance jewelry," "memorial jewelry," "miscarriage jewelry," "stillbirth jewelry," "infant loss jewelry," or "baby loss jewelry." You will commonly find items that feature birthstones and religious references like angels. Choose what resonates for you. If you have physical remains from your womb loss, such as ashes, you might search "cremation jewelry" for options that can incorporate them. If you would like to use jewelry you already have, perhaps clean it physically or leave it out to be cleansed energetically by the sunlight or moonlight. Once you have a piece of jewelry in hand, close your eyes and think or say aloud your intention for it, imbuing it with your meaning and making it sacred. You can wear and touch this jewelry in a ritualistic way or whenever you need something physical to help you feel anchored in the present moment. In addition to or instead of jewelry, perhaps consider other ways to memorialize your grief and resilience with your body, such as tattoos. If having something on your body doesn't feel right, perhaps consider another remembrance item, such as a reborn doll. Whatever you choose, may it be an item that feels most true to you and your needs, comforting when you see it, and grounding when you touch it.

Self-Tending Heals Us All

As you honor your body, your needs, and your grief, you show the world that womb loss survivors are worth tending to. You help heal the collective through your example, and you help others see what is possible for them. You may also feel called to do more to support the womb loss community. This was true for me and how this book came to be. I wanted others to know what I wish I had known and to feel what I wish I had felt. Tending to the community can look many different ways. It can be as simple as offering someone a small gesture of care you would have wanted for yourself, like a hug, a gift certificate for meal delivery, or a condolence card that communicates the sentiment, "I see you hurting, and I am with you." You may only be able to focus on yourself right now or ever, and that's okay too. However you feel drawn to tending, know that your loving intention creates ripples that help soothe and hold us all—for your loss is our loss, and your healing is our healing.

The following practice is an invitation to hold space for other womb loss survivors.

GROUNDING RELATIONAL PRACTICE

Hosting a Gathering for Womb Loss Survivors

Even if we don't see what we need reflected in our world, know, dear reader, that we can create a new culture of compassion for womb loss and those of us who experience it. It begins with self-tending, and as we experience the power of centering and honoring ourselves, may we help others know the same.

The Invitation

I began this book describing how it emerged from the Our Womb Loss dining events I hosted in Los Angeles, centering and honoring those who, like me, had endured pregnancy and infant loss. I invite you to gather in a similar way with others who know womb loss as we do. The intention here is simply to be in community with other womb loss survivors to honor yourselves and one another. This can look many ways, and you are welcome to manifest what feels right for you. You might host a small gathering in your home, meet at a restaurant, or connect virtually. The following is a general outline of the dining events I've hosted. You are welcome to reference it or intuit your own way.

1. Invite your community to gather for an afternoon or evening to honor themselves and their experience of pregnancy and infant loss. The invitation can be as casual as a text message or an email. As with

any event invitation, state the basic information, such as the date, the start and end times, the address, and a short description explaining the intention for the gathering.

2. Offer your community and yourself a moment to deepen your connection before eating. This can include welcoming everyone, then taking turns to share your names and what drew each of you to be there, each person sharing only as much as feels right for them. During this time, invite attendees to simply listen and hold space for the one talking. You might then transition to the meal by thanking everyone for showing up for themselves and one another to honor your collective grief.

3. Nourish your community and yourself with postpartum foods to honor that you, too, are postpartum after pregnancy and infant loss. If you are meeting online, you might invite everyone to come prepared with a dish or drink for themselves. Let this time naturally invite more conversation amongst attendees, helping them connect to a tangible sense of community.

4. Integrate a ritual of self-tending after the meal, which might be any of the practices shared in this book. It can be as simple as presenting a tray of candles (electric or wax) and inviting each guest to take a candle for themselves and each of their losses. Then, invite guests to light the candles and sit with them for a moment of silence or against the backdrop of a meaningful song. Invite attendees to turn off or blow out their candles when they feel ready, and perhaps ask everyone to offer some words of reflection.

5. Bring the gathering to a close by thanking everyone for showing up for themselves and one another, and encourage attendees to be gentle with themselves as they transition back into their lives.

Offering from the Collective

The following is an offering from two women I hold near and dear. Kiley and Betsy are the heart and soul behind the nonprofit organization Return to Zero: HOPE, an organization I noted earlier that provides compassionate support for anyone touched by pregnancy and infant loss. Their offerings include holistic retreats for bereaved mothers that tend deeply to their bodies, needs, and grief. Being present at two of these retreats has given me such an appreciation for the power of community. To be in a beautiful place surrounded by nature and others who know womb loss with their bodies is hard to put into words fully. It is like coming home. You leave knowing what kind of support is possible for us, what we deserve, and how much it is needed in the world.

AN OFFERING BY KILEY KREKORIAN HANISH
AND BETSY WINTER

Support Groups and Retreats

What it is

For those who have experienced pregnancy and infant loss, support groups and retreats offer the opportunity to make connections in a brave and sacred environment with others who have been through a similar experience. There are various support groups and retreats, virtual or in person, for free or for a fee (some on a sliding scale). Support groups are usually led by a facilitator who is knowledgeable or has personal experience with perinatal loss. Some adhere to a drop-in structure, while others are closed groups that last for several weeks or months. They can consist of open discussion with little facilitation or be highly structured and education-based. Retreats are usually more immersive, with shared community experiences lasting one to a few days, and are hosted somewhere that helps attendees feel they are retreating from their daily lives for that short period.

How it can support you

Pregnancy and infant loss is a type of loss that can feel very isolating, and yet, humans are social beings with the inherent need to feel witnessed and held in both our joy and sorrow. Finding the right support helps you know you are not alone. Support groups and retreats centered around the shared experience of pregnancy and infant loss create a sense of community that is essential to grieving and healing. They can help bereaved parents process their emotions, integrate their loss, gain greater self-understanding, and develop deep, lasting friendships that carry them through the ups and downs of grieving, postpartum healing, and all that is to come. In these spaces, you can show up as you are without hiding the parts that are hurting.

A Gentle Hand

A self-tending practice

Find a quiet, comfortable space and take a moment to ask yourself how you are feeling in this moment. As you identify what you are feeling, you might also notice where you are experiencing this feeling in your body. If you notice multiple feelings, you might choose one to focus on for now. Notice how the feeling is finding its voice through your body. Give yourself permission to feel the sensations for a moment. You can rest a hand compassionately on the area where the sensation is strongest, receiving your hand's kind presence through your skin and sensing its support from the inside out. You might then invite your breath into this area. Is it possible to breathe kindness, grace, and compassion into this part of yourself? What do you notice when you really feel into this gentle hand that is alongside whatever is coming up for you? Allow yourself to feel felt, felt by the loving presence of your own hand, and know you can offer yourself your own compassionate presence at any time.

A Gentle Closing

Thank you for being here. For showing up for yourself, your body, and your grief as we explored how to support survivors of womb loss—you and those around you. As we tend to our needs, we model what healing after womb loss can look like. And as we tend to others who have endured this pain, we help create the world we deserve. One that acknowledges us and our loss, that knows how to hold us, and that knows how to tend to us. May you be gentle with yourself as you tend to your needs, remembering that there is a community here for you. That, in fact, community is essential to our individual healing and that you do not have to endure this alone.

As this chapter comes to a close, I invite you to pause for a few breaths and with the closing verse to help you transition gently back into your life or to the next part of the book. And if anything in this chapter activated a strong response, consider doing something more to feel grounded. This may be an act of self-tending or reaching out to someone you trust for support. Honor what you need in this moment.

I am here, as I am.
And so it is.

You are here.
And we are with you.

CHAPTER 10

Returning and Becoming

This is your process. Take your time.

I n 2015, the world came to know of a gorilla named Shira, who carried the body of her dead, week-old baby around her enclosure at Frankfurt Zoo in Germany. Shira was reluctant to let her go and desperate to wake her up.[1] It was her second baby and her second infant loss. In 2018, a killer whale named Tahlequah captured the attention and hearts of people all over the world as she swam for over two weeks while carrying the body of her dead calf, continually nudging the body toward the surface of the Pacific Ocean to keep her baby from sinking.[2] To see such grief among other mammals illustrates the universal heartbreak womb loss brings. It also affirms the primal need to feel a tangible connection to our womb loss. It normalizes the desire to touch and hold the body, the remains, with tenderness and to process the loss in our own time and in our own way.

~

As you begin to consider returning to your life after birthing loss and your process of becoming someone whom the loss has changed, may stories such as these help you trust yourself, your animal body, and your intuition.

Considering the Future

It is common for the experience of womb loss to bring into question many aspects of our being. As we begin to return to our lives, we may find that what felt right to us before our loss no longer feels aligned. This is understandable since womb loss has the power to change us deeply and irrevocably. You may no longer resonate with your work or certain relationships. Parts of your own identity may be in flux. For example, "How many children do you have?" or "Do you have kids?" are questions we may hear that prompt us to think about our identity as a parent. If you do not have living children, do you consider yourself a mother? A parent? Your response may shift over time or depend on who is asking and the context of that interaction. In the years since my pregnancy losses, my answer has shifted. Recently, I have felt compelled to say, "I have three living children," adding the adjective "living" to bring awareness to the fact that I have two children who are not. Sometimes, people notice, and the conversation will unfold further. Sometimes, people seem to catch the nuance but choose not to ask about it.

As you transition back into your life, you may realize you want or need changes to happen but are unsure what exactly, and that's okay. In such moments, you can return to the simplicity and constancy of your breath and allow yourself time to gain the clarity you seek.

While much of this book is about being in the present moment and honoring what feels right to you now, it can also be helpful to think about the future and how you want to feel then. The following practice is an invitation to consider your hopes for the future, knowing that what you feel now may not always be your reality.

GROUNDING BREATHING PRACTICE

Breathing into the Future

Sometimes, it can be hard to be in the present moment with our grief and to be in our bodies after pregnancy and birth have changed it. Sometimes, we need a break from our grief and the discomfort and pain in our bodies. If the current moment feels too hard to be in, that is understandable and okay. Take a moment to think about your future and what you want for it instead. Offer yourself solace as you imagine and feel into a different experience for yourself.

The Invitation

When you are ready, find a comfortable resting position seated or lying down, perhaps with a blanket to give you warmth and a sense of protection. If seated, you might rest your hands over your heart or in your lap. If lying down, you might choose to rest your hands over your womb or simply let your arms rest along the sides of your body. You are welcome to close your eyes or soften your gaze as you allow your mind to focus gently on your breathing. Then, taking your time, begin to think about how you want to feel in the future. Allow a word or words to emerge intuitively, and choose one that resonates most strongly for you in this moment. Once you have chosen a word, you can say it silently or aloud with each breath. Allow it to be a mantra for your healing. Allow yourself to embody the word as if you are feeling it now in truth. You can continue breathing this way for as long as you like. When you are ready, you can take a deep cleansing breath to help you transition back into the room and open your eyes if they are closed.

Remember Our Beginning

As you transition back into parts of your life and as you remake others, including your own identity, it can be helpful to consider what comforted us when we were young. Everyone on earth comes from the same place: someone's womb. Despite all that divides us, we have this first home in common. Let us remember what we and every single human feels in our first months of existence, knowing we can return to those primal elements of comfort as we continue our grieving and postpartum healing journey: warmth; gentle, consistent touch and movement; nourishment; soothing darkness; and connection with another human being. What comforted us then can comfort us now. Think, too, of what felt comforting to you through your childhood and consider how you might weave those experiences into your grieving and postpartum healing processes. As adults, it is rare to be tended to as dearly as we were as babies and children. And yet, what comforted us then can comfort us now.

The following practice is an invitation to take a break from tending to your grief directly by returning to a fond memory. This can help remind you that what you feel now is not the only way you can feel.

A Place You Miss

The Invitation

You are welcome to begin in any comfortable resting position, either seated or lying down, perhaps draping a blanket over yourself to keep you warm and safely cocooned. Allow your awareness to gently focus on your breath, letting it follow each inhalation and exhalation as you settle into rest. When you are ready, I invite you to think of a place you have visited that you miss, somewhere you would like to return and that brings fond memories. Let this place emerge in your consciousness rather than trying to think of one, and explore your memory of this place using all your senses. You might recall what you saw there, what you smelled, what you tasted, what you heard, and what you touched. How did you feel when you were there? Perhaps sit with this last question for a moment, allowing yourself to feel now what you felt then, knowing such felt experiences are stored in your body. When you are ready to bring this practice to a close, take a deep cleansing breath and slowly stretch your arms and legs to help you transition gently.

Ever-Present, Ever-Shifting Grief

As you continue grieving and healing from womb loss, you may find that over time your grief changes, just as your life changes. You may always feel a sense of grief, but how it feels may shift. Keeping this in mind may help in moments when your grief feels intense and overwhelming. How you feel is valid, and how you feel can change. It may soften. It may include more fond memories than traumatic ones. It may transform into energy that helps you do healing work in the world. Your grief may be ever present, but it may not always feel the way it does today.

The following practice is an invitation to pause and reflect on your grief over time to see what shifts may have happened already. I often use it when leading grief support groups and have witnessed how powerful this simple practice can be. I share it here with permission from Our House Grief Support Center in Los Angeles.

Yesterday, Today, Tomorrow

Grieving is a process, just as returning to your life in a postbirth, postloss body is a process. Just as becoming a different version of you after grief is a process. Please honor how your unique process unfolds with kindness, patience, and love. You will need paper and something to write with. You can also have art supplies like colored pencils ready, but this is optional.

The Invitation

Find your way into a comfortable seated position, taking a moment to breathe deeply or press down into the parts of you touching the earth to help you feel grounded in the present moment. Then, when you are ready, I invite you to fold your paper into three sections or draw lines to divide it into thirds. Label the left section "Yesterday," the middle section "Today," and the right section "Tomorrow." Reflect on your grief yesterday or further in the past, and fill in the left section of your paper with words and images that describe it. Next, take some time to reflect on how your grief feels today, and fill the middle section with words and/or images. Finally, what do you hope your grief will be like tomorrow or further in the future? Add words and images to represent your thoughts in the right section. Take a moment to sit with what landed on the page.

Nurturing Jujube Tonic

A Recipe by Heng Ou and Marisa Belger

We are constantly in transition, especially in our culture, which values doing over being. I think this is why it can be so comforting to feel grounded and held. The following is a nourishing recipe meant to hold you through your transitions. It is by two women who are very special to me: Heng Ou, who has supported my efforts to tend to womb loss survivors since the beginning and who tended to me during my pregnancies, and Marisa Belger, who has held space for me as a book coach and motherhood coach. They are authors of *The First Forty Days: The Essential Art of Nourishing the New Mother,* which helped bring postpartum care into wider consciousness in the US. I am honored that they can be present for you through this recipe.

~

Jujubes, a stone fruit harvested in the fall and highly valued in Chinese medicine, are particularly beneficial for recovery after blood loss, womb loss, or menstruation. Rich in antioxidants and vitamin C, they aid the body's healing and serve as an excellent elixir for immune health. Their calming properties promote restful sleep, which is crucial for postpartum healing and grieving.

When combined with raspberry leaves, known for enhancing uterine health, jujubes create a nurturing tonic. This blend offers a thoughtful, holistic approach to postpartum recovery after womb loss, providing both physical and emotional support. Sip this tonic slowly and reflect on the thoughts or feelings that arise. It's a soft, feminine tonic, designed to serve and support your needs during transitional times.

- 8 cups water
- 16 dried jujubes
- 2 cinnamon sticks or 1 teaspoon of cinnamon powder
- 1/2 cup raspberry leaves

In a medium pot, bring water to a light boil. Rinse and tear the jujubes in half, keeping the seed intact as it helps relax the body. Add jujubes and cinnamon to the pot and cook over medium heat. After simmering for 30 minutes, reduce the heat to medium-low.

Once the tea turns a darker brown and the water level has reduced by about an inch, turn off the heat. Add the raspberry leaves, cover the pot, and allow it to steep for 20 minutes. Strain and squeeze out any remaining liquid from the jujubes. Enjoy warm.

Returning to Our Bodies

Our life experiences leave impressions on our bodies and spirits. Some lighter. Some deeper. Some impressions feel comforting and uplifting; others we would rather not feel. Traumatic impressions from womb loss can continue to be held in the body, making it difficult to relax. Physical reminders of pregnancy, such as a pronounced belly, may be hard to live with and also lead to people asking if you are pregnant or when you are due. This may activate strong feelings and memories of your loss. In places like the US, there is great pressure to "bounce back" after pregnancy, and you may feel this too. You may feel this pressure even more without a living baby to show for your efforts. It can be incredibly hard to be in our bodies during and after womb loss, and yet our bodies are our forever homes. We are worthy of living in our homes with comfort and ease. Returning to your body may be a slow process, and that's okay. It may begin by simply noticing sensations or with a single yoga pose, with gentle touch from ourselves or someone we trust, or with kind words. The following is a compassionate phrase I often say to myself when I struggle to feel at home in my body: "This is where I'm at." Saying this helps me acknowledge that I may not feel the way I want in my body, *and* where I am right now is okay. Please be gentle and patient with your postpartum, postloss body. It has been through so much.

The following practice is an invitation to move intuitively as you allow your thoughts to quiet and your body a chance to speak.

GROUNDING EMBODIMENT PRACTICE

Let Your Body Tell Its Story

Moving intuitively to music that is meaningful to you may elicit strong feelings and felt sensations. You may even feel an urge to cry. As you have done throughout this book, please honor what you need in any given moment, allowing yourself to take breaks or stop altogether. Remember that everything here is an invitation, and you get to choose what to do. You will need a song (or playlist of songs) that resonates with your grief, comfortable clothing you can easily move in, a yoga mat or blanket, and candles (optional).

The Invitation

When you are ready, find a quiet space to be alone for at least fifteen minutes. You might adjust the space to create a womblike environment, such as lowering window coverings if it is daytime, dimming lights, or using candlelight. If the floor is hard, you might create a soft place to land by laying down a yoga mat or blanket.

Find your way into a comfortable seated position on the ground with your legs crossed, knees bent, and feet tucked under. If you have chosen one song, you might set it on repeat so that it plays for the duration of your movement. Take a deep breath or two, then begin playing your chosen music. Soften your gaze or close your eyes as you listen to the music playing, and place the palms of your hands over your knees. Allow your heart to guide your chest into a gentle forward tilt, a posture that honors the natural collapse of grief. Then, take your time as you move the upper body to the right, to the back, and the left, slowly creating circles as you hold on to your knees for support. You are welcome to continue moving this way for as long as it feels right for you, perhaps pausing in areas where you'd like to feel a deeper stretch or rounding the shoulders forward whenever you lean back. Then, switch directions when you are ready. Allow this movement to gently warm your body and invite a transition from a thinking state to an intuitive state.

Allow your body to lead. Your body may want to explore more movement seated, maybe reaching one arm to the sky and letting the other follow. Maybe moving onto hands and knees into Polar Bear or Child's Pose or lying on the ground while your limbs move freely. Perhaps your body wants to slowly make its way to a wall, placing your hands on the wall and feeling its solid presence as you come to stand. Maybe your body wants to explore walking slowly around the space, letting your feet feel the floor and your hands feel the objects around you. If you find yourself thinking about what to do next, allow your mind to focus on the sounds of the music and the sensations as you move. This moment is for your body. What does your body need to say? What stories does your body want to share? When you are ready to bring this practice to a close, you can come into stillness, return your awareness to your breath, and slowly open your eyes if they are closed.

If moving intuitively is new to you, it may feel uncomfortable, awkward, or even silly. However you feel about it is okay. You might return to this practice later and notice if it feels any different. As you continue to explore intuitive movement, let your body be the guide and honor what it needs. May your mind and body feel more aligned, and may such integration offer you some relief.

Pregnancy After Loss (Or Not)

The experience of pregnancy is so different after you have known womb loss. What I know from personal experience and have witnessed in many others is that anxiety and fear can be ever present, tempering any excitement and wearing on all levels of our being. Not only are you grieving your previous womb loss(es), but you may also feel *anticipatory grief,* typically described as grief that is felt before a loss.[3] It is hard not to worry that womb loss will occur again, hard not to worry that the next day will bring symptoms of loss or that the next appointment will bring heartbreaking news. It can be difficult to relax and feel joy when you know full well the risks involved in pregnancy and how much about the process is out of your hands. It can feel like you are holding your breath until the birth of yet another loss or a living child. It is hard to be pregnant after loss, *and* it is possible to endure, though it may feel like you are getting by just one day at a time or even one moment at a time. You are not alone in feeling this. Many of us understand. There is so much more that can be said about this topic that an entire book can be written about it, and one such book exists: *Rebirth: The Journey of Pregnancy After a Loss* by Joey Miller, MSW, LCSW. Consider referring to this valuable resource if you are pregnant after womb loss.

The following practice is an invitation to honor your individual and shared journey of womb loss with a simple ritual for you and your loved ones. Honoring the loss(es) you have experienced can help soften difficult feelings that arise in subsequent pregnancies. And for those who cannot or choose not to get pregnant again, honoring the end of your fertility journey is just as important. The closing of this chapter in your life deserves your attention and tending. I hope the following ritual can support you in honoring this threshold and all the layers of feeling that may accompany it.

Candles for All

Rituals like this and all those included in this book can help you honor threshold moments with an act that is infused with loving intention. They can help you pause and honor smaller moments as well as major ones. Rituals are a way to declare that you, this moment, and what this moment means to you are worth acknowledging. May this ritual offer healing acknowledgment for you and all who have been touched by your loss. You will need candles (electric or wax)—one for each person present and one for each womb loss.

The Invitation

Welcome your loved ones to join you for this ritual. If you are partnered or have living children, consider inviting them to participate. Set your candles on a surface such as a dining or remembrance table. When you are ready, light one candle at a time, following the suggested script below. You might feel called to say more after you light each candle or to use your own words altogether. That is completely okay and supported. Let your intuition guide you and honor what feels right for you in this moment.

- Light the first candle and say, "I light this candle in honor of me and all I have been through."

- Continue lighting the candles, one for each person present, saying, "I light this candle in honor of you, [name of person], and all you have been through."

- Light the remaining candle(s), saying, "I light this candle in honor of our womb loss/baby," or, "I light these candles in honor of our womb losses/babies." If applicable, you can share the name of each baby you are honoring as you light their candle.

- Once all the candles are lit, you might take a moment to sit and gaze at them in silence. When you are ready to bring this practice to a close, blow out the candles together.

~

This is a variation of a ritual I often do with my postpartum doula clients in our last session. It is a simple yet powerful way to honor our time together and bring it to a clear and gentle close. In its original version, I light a candle in honor of the mother or gestating parent and share a few sentences to reflect on the challenges they faced and the resilience they embodied. I light the second candle in honor of their partner and share a few sentences to reflect on their journey and the support they've shown. Finally, I light a third candle in honor of their children, both living and deceased, and share a few sentences about the love their parents feel for them. Know that you are worthy of such acknowledgment, for you have endured so much and are enduring still.

Start Where You Are

Even if you are not where you want to be, allow yourself to start where you are. Tender things need time. Grieving and healing from womb loss can be a long, deeply felt process that remakes us. As my friend and acupuncturist Michelle Goebel-Angel once told me, "You have to root before you rise." Give yourself the gift of time, space, solitude, self-tending, and support to process your feelings so that you may honor the endings in front of you (end of a pregnancy, end of your fertility by choice or not, end of relationships, etc.) and feel rooted in your resilience before you rise back into the world anew.

The following practice is an invitation to connect with others in the loss community so that you may experience the medicine that feeling witnessed offers as you are in your process of returning and becoming. Feeling witnessed is an essential part of grieving and healing after pregnancy and infant loss. You are reminded that you are not alone and are reassured that what you feel is valid. Perhaps you will offer the same to another and experience the medicine that bearing witness also provides.

Connecting with the Loss Community

The Invitation

If and when it feels right for you, I invite you to connect with at least one other person in the womb loss community. You might reach out to an organization like the Pregnancy and Infant Loss Support Centre. Although based in Canada, PILSC offers free and confidential services for anyone in the world. This includes text or online chat services, virtual one-on-one support from their certified counselors, pregnancy-and-infant-loss coaches, peer mentors, and support groups. You might also refer to the website of the US-based nonprofit organization Return to Zero: HOPE, which has an extensive pregnancy-and-infant-loss directory that includes national and international organizations and providers. Or you might connect with someone in your social circle who has experienced pregnancy and infant loss.

If this feels daunting or difficult in any way, you are welcome to come back to this invitation at a later time, if at all. You can make this practice your own by finding another way to feel connected to someone else who has experienced womb loss, maybe by reading a memoir or finding a pregnancy-and-infant-loss social media account to follow. However you build a connection with the womb loss community, may it be meaningful and genuinely helpful to your process of grieving and healing.

Offering from the Collective

The following is an offering from someone I greatly admire. Sparrow is a massage therapist and the owner of Sparrow's Nest in Los Angeles. A chance meeting and a twenty-minute neck and shoulder massage many years ago left a deep impression in the best way. Sparrow immediately came to mind as I thought about who could share heartfelt words and wisdom in this book. Sparrow's grounded presence, kind spirit, and healing hands are memorable; these attributes come through in her center's offerings. One such offering is unique because it is not widely known or offered:

bereavement postpartum massage. I was pleasantly surprised to see this on her website as an explicit offering with its own page. Sparrow and I agree that massage that is sensitive to our needs as both postpartum and bereaved is needed—that it is, in fact, essential.

AN OFFERING BY SPARROW HARRINGTON

Bereavement Massage

What it is

Bereavement massage is a postpartum massage with an added layer of emotional sensitivity. It can also be referred to as postpartum bereavement massage. Skilled, nurturing touch can benefit your physical recovery and emotional healing after any womb loss at any stage of gestation. I created this specific offering at Sparrow's Nest for women who did not find their exact situation reflected in our services. I wanted them to know that their unique needs deserve nurturing care too. I want all who experience womb loss to know that we see you and are honored to support you.

How it can support you

The bereaved body is still a postpartum body, so the same techniques we use to help our clients recover after birth are applicable here. This includes abdominal work to support the uterus as it returns to its pre-pregnancy size and to help organs return to their pre-pregnancy position. It also relieves musculoskeletal aches and pains, hormonal fluctuations, and pelvic pain common in a postpartum body. With the added reverence for your loss, bereavement massage can tend to the grief stored in the body and support the emotional processing of your womb loss. If your loss was medically uncomplicated, you may receive a bereavement massage right away or as soon as you feel ready. Know that it is never too late to receive a bereavement massage. Whether it's been weeks, months, or years since your loss, grieving and healing are not linear. If you feel you would benefit from this type of physical nurturing, please honor that urge and know that you deserve to feel held and tended to. If your loss involved complications like surgery or hemorrhaging, please defer to your care provider to clear you for massage and communicate any recommended modifications to your massage therapist.

Postloss Self-Massage for Your Sacred Womb

A self-tending practice

These instructions provide a gentle and nurturing womb massage routine after womb loss. Remember to listen to your body and adjust the pressure and movements as needed for comfort. If your womb is too tender to touch right now, that is okay. Consider returning to this self-tending practice if and when you feel ready.

1. Find a comfortable place: Find a quiet and warm place to lie down comfortably.

2. Heat your belly (optional): Lie belly-down on a heating pad for 5 to 10 minutes to warm your womb before starting.

3. Prepare your position: Lie on your back and place a pillow under your knees for support.

4. Use a heating pad (optional): You can place the heating pad underneath your lower back during the massage.

5. Position your hands: Place your hands over your womb, which is located below your navel and above your pubic bone. Don't worry about being precise; the goal is to connect with this sacred space and breathe. Acknowledge any emotions that come to the surface. What is your womb holding? If there's rage or grief or a sense that your body betrayed you, acknowledge that, and then, if you're open to it, see if you're willing to shift. Ask yourself if you're willing to be on the same team as your body, even if it's just a hint of willingness or curiosity. Breathe.

6. Set an intention: Create an intention for this time with your womb. It may be to connect with your womb with gentleness. It may be to nurture this sacred place that held life or to forgive and rebuild trust in your body.

7. Apply massage oil: Take a quarter-sized amount of oil (like organic fractionated coconut oil) and rub it between your hands until there is a subtle glistening of oil across the palms and fingertips.

8. Begin the massage: Place your oiled hands on your abdomen (belly), starting with the entire abdomen and then focusing more specifically on your womb.

9. Move clockwise: Begin by moving your hands in a clockwise direction, following the natural orientation of your intestines. Use broad, sweeping strokes, ensuring your hands are light, soft, and gentle. Allow them to mold to the shape of your torso. Create a clockwise circle, starting from under your ribs, sweeping down the side of your body, going above your pubic bone, and then back around again. You can use both hands, with one hand following the other in the same clockwise pattern, or you may choose to use just your dominant hand for this movement.

10. Draw energy to your center: After a few minutes of warming and circling, gently move your hands from the outermost sides of your abdomen, following the path between your ribs and the ilium (hip bone), and sweep them toward your center, aiming for your midline or your umbilicus (belly button). This helps draw your energy and focus back to your center after the expansive experience of pregnancy and loss.

11. Create triangle formation: Form an upside-down triangle with your hands by placing the tips of your two thumbs together and connecting your index fingers. Position this triangle with the base over your belly button and the center of the triangle over your womb (which lies underneath it).

12. Stationary circles: While keeping your hands in the triangle formation, create small stationary circles over your womb space. You can gently press down toward your back and lift your womb toward your belly button, then lower it back to its original position.

13. Side-to-side movement: Press down an inch or two toward your back and gently move your fingers side to side, rocking your womb back and forth. Repeat this with diagonal lifts on the right and left sides, focusing more time on any areas that feel tight or imbalanced.

14. Promote flow and connection: The massage aims to create movement, flow, circulation, and connection in this area, and in doing so, it draws your energy back into your center, nurturing your sacred womb.

15. Finish with broad strokes: Finish the massage by returning to broad clockwise strokes over your whole belly, closing the session, and thanking your body for this opportunity to reconnect. Over time, with continuous and gentle tending, you can build rapport and trust with your body. You may also consider receiving a postpartum bereavement massage or a traditional closing of the bones ceremony for further support.

A Gentle Closing

Thank you for being here. For showing up for yourself, your body, and your grief as we explored more considerations for your time after birthing your womb loss. These included shifts in your identity, how you show up to your life, and how the postpartum time after womb loss is both a returning and becoming—returning to parts of your life as it was before your loss and becoming what you need now. May you be gentle with yourself and remember that this is your process and you can take your time.

As this chapter comes to a close, I invite you to pause for a few breaths and with the closing verse to help you transition gently back into your life or to the next part of the book. And if anything in this chapter activated a strong response, consider doing something more to feel grounded. This may be an act of self-tending or reaching out to someone you trust for support. Honor what you need in this moment.

I am here, as I am.
And so it is.

You are here.
And we are with you.

Letter from the Author

Dearest reader,

Thank you for being here with me alongside countless others who know womb loss in and with our bodies. *And* I wish you didn't have reason to be here with us—that you could have known the beauty of pregnancy without the pain of loss.

I have spent the past seven years grieving my womb losses, feeling what they mean to me. I have spent the past seven years mourning my womb losses, sharing what they mean to me by holding space for others like us. I want us all to know that we too give birth, we too are postpartum, and we too deserve tending. We also deserve to have our loss acknowledged and our grief validated and to feel held as we grieve and mourn through the hours, days, weeks, months, years, and decades. I have spent the past four years writing this book from a deeply embodied place, where my grief feels poignant still, so that you may feel the vibration of my grief and know you are not alone.

Remember, there is no set way or timeline for tending to your grief. Grieving and postpartum healing are nonlinear processes that depend greatly on your body, your needs, and your context. Maybe it was hard to acknowledge your loss fully when it occurred, and it is only now, many years later, that you are remembering. That's okay. You get to go at your own pace. You get to choose when to turn toward your grief. When to face your grief. When to step toward your grief. When to lean into your grief. And maybe one day, when to embrace this part of you in a warm hug.

As our time together comes to an end, I would like to share one more story. In the summer of 2022, my family and I stayed just outside the eastern entrance of Zion National Park on the traditional land of the Ancestral Puebloans and Southern Paiute. With only a few other RVs nearby and forty acres of untouched desert around us, it was a welcome respite from our usual way of living. One night, as my husband prepared the fire pit for our living children to make smores, I stepped out of our Airstream trailer and looked up. It was as if time stopped. I took in the darkest sky I had ever seen, blanketed with the brightest stars I had ever laid my eyes on. I turned in a slow circle, absorbing the moment. I felt like I was standing in a dark snow globe with stars floating all around me. My awe deepened as I considered the years it took for the starlight to reach me. Then I felt sadness because it wasn't until my late thirties that I was seeing the night sky in its natural state, its beauty unencumbered by light pollution. *This has always been here,* I thought to myself.

And this is how I feel about our resilience—yours and mine. Even if life experiences and trauma have made it hard to see, within each of us is an inherent resilience. Ever present and radiant like the stars in a dark sky. May you know this and trust in your resilience to hold you through these trying and tender times.

Please be gentle with yourself, dear reader. Be gentle with your grief, your trauma, your postpartum body. And may you live gently. One day at a time. One moment at a time. One breath at a time.

I end with caring words from my beloved friend Molly Boeder Harris, who has a way with language that never fails to nourish me: *Sending love, gentleness, and all the soothing scents, nourishing foods, warm drinks, supportive movement, and tender physical contact that can hold you through these painful days.*

From my depths to yours,

Eileen

Letter from the Artist

Dear ones,

I offer you this bouquet of deeply healing florals and herbs for your womb loss and for your health. I offer you this creation with all of my heart, drawing upon my own journey through motherhood, years of postpartum depression, and the profound healing I feel when I put ink to paper.

When Eileen asked me to illustrate her book over three years ago, I was incredibly moved and honored to hold space for her vision. The cover art soon became *our* vision as we co-created during hikes in the canyons, shared meals, tears, and conversations. I sat with my intentions for connecting with you, dear reader, for a long time—usually vibrating with energy after spending hours with Eileen. I knew I wanted to create art that was sensitive and thoughtful to the loss you have experienced and to evoke a deep well of ancestral wisdom, calling upon waves of powerful women all around you—past, present, and future.

While daydreaming of how to honor the womb, *she* started coming to me—the rich bouquet that you see on the cover—asking to be offered to you just as we would offer flowers to anyone grieving a loss, a death, or other painful transition. This bouquet contains multitudes—divine plant medicine that has the collective energy to recognize, heal, uplift, inspire, cocoon, nourish, and strengthen.

Beginning with Osmanthus for peace, self-healing, and fertility. Wild and abundant in Kaiping, China, where I spent my earliest years, I am returned to the comforting energy of my beginnings whenever I smell her subtle, fuzzy apricot notes. Ylang-ylang to soothe and lift one's mood. With roots in the Philippines, she honors part of Eileen's ethnic heritage and helps her feel held.

Wild California rose for self-love, compassion, and softening of the heart. She anchors the bottom center of the bouquet and pays homage to our shared home here in California on Tongva and Acjachemen ancestral land. Motherwort, likened to a gentle, maternal hug, can be found in my mother's carefully tended garden. Cacao for opening the heart and easing the weight it carries. Sacred and medicinal to many South American cultures, she is said to carry the essence of the feminine and also offers a loving, motherly presence. Sweetgrass, a sacred medicine of the Indigenous cultures of North America; her smoke is used to cleanse and protect the body. Vanilla (which comes from the Latin word *vagina*!) for warmth and simplicity. Dates to support labor and build strength. Jasmine for motherhood, respect, and beauty. Saffron for cleansing, integration, and protection. Jujubes for rest and digestion. And eucalyptus for resilience. In all of this, I wanted *our* uterus to be lush and evocative of our collective spirit: complex, resilient, and perfectly imperfect. Soft *and* strong. Beautiful.

These same plants are gently scattered across the illustrations within the book, as if the cover art were carried on a breeze to eventually return to the earth, to become dust, to become new life. Floating in the space above is a pulsating orb of light—perhaps a sunrise, a sunset, or an invitation to what's possible. Layered under the inkwork is a wave of earth tones, grounding you and evoking the iron hues of our body's most sacred fluid.

I hope my art can help you breathe into the deepest and most tender love for yourself and that you see your sacred womb mirrored back.

With love,

Meaningful Dates

- First Sunday in May ~ International Bereaved Mother's Day
- July ~ Bereaved Parents Awareness Month
- Last Sunday in August ~ International Bereaved Father's Day
- First Sunday after Labor Day in September ~ Grandparents' Day
- October ~ Pregnancy and Infant Loss Awareness Month
- October 15 ~ Pregnancy and Infant Loss Remembrance Day
- October 15 at 7:00 pm local time ~ International Wave of Light
- November ~ Worldwide Bereaved Siblings Month

You are invited to use the space below to add and honor any dates that are meaningful to you and your unique experience of womb loss.

A Closing Blessing
for the Postpartum and Bereaved

May you feel seen.
May you feel heard.
May you feel held.

And in times when you do not, may you know that you are deserving of all these things.

May you be grounded.
May you be slow.
May you be gentle.

And in times when you are not, may you return to your breath and simply be.

May you know your body.
May you know a softer way of being.
May you know your worth.

And in times when that is hard, may you choose yourself over others, even if only for a moment.

Acknowledgments

To Joelle Hann of Brooklyn Book Doctor and my Book Proposal Academy colleagues. It was an intense six months of weekly Zoom calls and writing our way through the first months of the COVID-19 pandemic. Our group was a sacred container, helping me to stay grounded and connected to something meaningful amidst the unraveling happening around us. I could not have finished my book proposal so swiftly without you, and I look back with awe at what we accomplished during the trauma of that time. *I thank you. I appreciate you.*

To Randee Braham of Noble Shit Consulting and Natalie Alcala of Fashion Mamas. It was because of a post in our Fashion Mamas Facebook group that I found my way to my dream literary agent. Thank you, Natalie, for creating and sustaining such an amazing community of creative mother entrepreneurs; and thank you, Randee, for your generosity. *I thank you. I appreciate you.*

To my literary agent, Zoe Sandler. We found each other in such a divine way, and I couldn't have asked for a better advocate for this book. You resonated with my book proposal from a deep and raw place, and I knew the first time we spoke that you were meant to be part of this journey with me. And what a perfect book doula you have been! You have held me through the years of my book's gestation, through the months as I labored to bring it all together in a cohesive form, through those challenging weeks of revisions when the pain felt so much like transition, and finally as I birthed it. Through all of this, you became a trusted friend I can turn to with both my wins and woes. Though your babies are not here physically, their presence is still felt, and powerfully so, as they helped usher this book into the world. I am forever grateful to you, dear Zoe, and I am look forward to what we do next. *I thank you. I appreciate you.*

To my editor, Haven Iverson. As with Zoe, our paths crossed in what felt like a powerful moment of alignment. You, too, resonated with my book proposal in a deep way that only someone who knows womb loss in their body can. And while so many were reluctant to take on this sensitive subject matter, you were ardent in your desire to help other womb loss survivors with this book. It ended up taking me four years to write as another pregnancy, another birth, another postpartum period, several deaths, and surviving a global pandemic took precedence. The entire time, you received me with warmth, understood my struggles as a working mother, and reassured me time and time again that everything would be okay. You have held both me and the spirit of this book in your tender embrace all these years, midwifing me so I could birth my book baby, feeling unquestionably supported. I am forever changed, in the best of ways, because of our relationship, and the world will know this book because you advocated so tirelessly for it and me. Thank you for revisiting such a painful part of your life to hold space for this book from an embodied place. Though unable to be here in the flesh, your baby's presence is felt through our work together—their legacy is a powerful one you can be so proud of. *I thank you. I appreciate you.*

To Tami Simon and the team at Sounds True. Little did I know in all the years of reading your books that I would one day have the honor of being part of your family of writers. It is a dream to be among the wise ones who have come before. Your team believed in me and my book as the topic of pregnancy and infant loss was just beginning to gain widespread attention. It felt ahead of its time as publisher after publisher passed on my book proposal. When so many said, "No," you said, "Of course!" You believed in those of us who have endured this invisible trauma. You believed in the validity of our pain, our grief, and our needs as both postpartum and bereaved. In acquiring my book, you made a powerful commitment to help create a new culture of compassion for all who have experienced womb loss. I have felt seen, heard, and held by your team. I understand this is not the norm, and I am forever grateful to have found a publisher so wholeheartedly dedicated to co-creating and supporting the needs of a working mother like myself. Special thanks to the following people who offered such care to this book: Lisa Kerans, who took on the cover design with such sincere dedication to channeling the essence of this book; Vesela Simic, whose copyedits helped improve the manuscript immensely; and Sarosh, my sensitivity reader who offered invaluable feedback. Finally, special thanks to my amazing production editors, Joe Sweeney and Jade Lascelles, who helped transform my manuscript in Microsoft Word into the book you have now. To the entire Sounds True team: *I thank you. I appreciate you.*

To my artist, Jo Situ Allen. You, too, have held space for me and my book these past four years with patience and unwavering passion. I cherish our time together conceptualizing, researching, intuiting, word-smithing, and bearing witness to each other. Co-creating with a brown, Asian American woman was healing, as I saw myself reflected and felt affirmed in our shared life experiences. Thank you for feeling so deeply into the essence of my book and creating art that helps my readers know they deserve beauty. Powerful, sacred beauty. And that such beauty exists within them already. I'm so grateful we found each other through Fashion Mamas, and I'm excited for what we co-create next. *I thank you. I appreciate you.*

To all who shared offerings for the book. As I read each of your contributions, I felt my heart swell with gratitude to have you in my life as friends, healers, and colleagues. Each of your generous offerings is powerful on its own, but together, they embody a culture-shifting essence of love, compassion, and unapologetic tenderness that can't be denied. Thank you for modeling how all who support the pregnant and postpartum can tailor their services to honor the unique needs of womb loss survivors. You are helping to create a new world where grief and trauma-sensitive prenatal and postnatal care is the norm rather than the exception. Special thanks to the following individuals for reviewing portions of the manuscript and offering their invaluable professional insight: Atena Asiaii, MD, MPH, of the Freyja Clinic, whom I consulted for medical accuracy; Christine Mark-Griffin, LCSW, PMH-C, of the private therapy practice Spark All Wellness, whom I consulted for perinatal mood and anxiety disorders; Nicole Longmire, MPH,

IBCLC, PMH-C, of Mother Nurture, whom I consulted for information on lactation after loss; and Jane Austin of Jane Austin Yoga, whom I consulted for support with prenatal- and postpartum-appropriate yoga offerings. This book exists because each of you contributed not only your wisdom but also your love. *I thank you. I appreciate you.*

To Heng Ou, Kimberly Ann Johnson, and Marisa Belger. All three of you helped pave the way for my book with your books on postpartum care, and all three of you have held me in the most loving embrace through the years. Heng, thank you for believing in me and my vision for my Our Womb Loss dinners all those years ago and for becoming a dear and trusted part of my support network. You were essential in helping me through my fifth pregnancy amidst the pandemic, making the biweekly, two-plus-hour round-trip drive from Los Angeles to my home to bring me MotherBees food, which was beyond my expectations. I felt not only supported but also cherished, knowing you were willing to make that drive for me. At a time when I didn't have much contact with my usual support network, seeing you and feeling your consistent warm presence nourished me as much as your food did. Kimberly, thank you for your support as a healing practitioner after both of my early pregnancy losses and my subsequent pregnancies. I will always value the enthusiasm and support you shared as this book came to be. Marisa, thank you for being my book and life coach in the second year of my writing journey. It was because of you that I had the courage to ask for the extension I needed, and it was because of your compassion for my struggles as a mother that I learned how to talk to myself with more kindness. To all three of you: *I thank you. I appreciate you.*

To Our House Grief Support Center. It is an honor to be part of the Our House family, to support grievers as a group leader, and to feel supported by my fellow group leaders. Volunteering here has helped soften the edges of my grief and deepened my passion for creating a kinder, softer, grief-sensitive world. Special thanks to my longtime group supervisor, Dr. Joanne Weingarten—your warmth and wisdom all these years have left a deep impression on me that will continue to inform my work. To everyone at Our House: *I thank you. I appreciate you.*

To my loved ones who have supported me in my journey to manifest this book. Special thanks to my dearest friend Christine Raitt for hosting my Our Womb Loss dining events, which provided the genesis for this book. It is because of your generosity and unfailing support that this book is here. Special thanks to screenwriter and friend Natalie Antoci for the countless text messages and voice notes of emotional support. Words can't fully capture what you mean to me. I'm so glad our paths crossed at preschool drop-offs and pick-ups and that our relationship has deepened into such a loving, spiritual one. Because you held me, I was able to hold the vision for this book all these years. And finally, special thanks to my cousin Julie Munsayac for sharing your graphic design wisdom. Because of you, I was able to better communicate my vision for the book. To all of you who have held me with love, *I thank you. I appreciate you.*

To my family. Thank you to my husband, Roland, and my parents, Diana and Ron, for the support I needed to write this book, initially with two living children and then with three. It is because of your help with their care and schooling that I could step back and write. And last but certainly not least, thank you to my children. To my living children—Celine, Vera, and Dorian—for always being patient, understanding, and forgiving of me as I went through ups and downs with my writing. You embody the qualities our world needs more: understanding, forgiveness, vulnerability, and joyful curiosity. I am lucky to share my life with you. And to my two spirit babies—it is because of you that this book exists at all. Your physical time here was short, but your legacy is lasting. To my family: *I thank you. I appreciate you.*

Resources

The following is a curated list of resources. There are many more out there. May these be helpful stepping stones as you seek support for yourself and those who are enduring womb loss alongside you.

Books

Children's Books on Death, Grief, and Womb Loss

- *All from a Walnut*, Ammi-Joan Paquette and Felicita Sala
- *Always Sisters: A Story of Loss and Love*, Saira Mir and Shahrzad Maydani
- *Dear Star Baby*, Malcolm Newsome and Kamala Nair
- *A Kids Book About Grief*, Brennan C. Wood
- *Life and I: A Story About Death*, Elisabeth Helland Larsen and Marine Schneider

Death, Loss, and Grief

- *The Art of Grieving: Gentle Self-Care Practices to Heal a Broken Heart*, Corinne Laan
- *Holding Space: On Loving, Dying, and Letting Go*, Amy Wright Glenn
- *It's OK That You're Not OK: Meeting Grief and Loss in a Culture That Doesn't Understand*, Megan Devine

Pregnancy and Pregnancy After Loss

- *The Motherly Guide to Becoming Mama: Redefining the Pregnancy, Birth, and Postpartum Journey**, Jill Koziol and Liz Tenety with Diana Spalding, MSN, CNM

  *This pregnancy guide honors that not all pregnancies end in living children and includes an entire chapter on womb loss.

- *Rebirth: The Journey of Pregnancy After a Loss*, Joey Miller, MSW, LCSW

Pregnancy and Infant Loss

- *All the Love: Healing Your Heart and Finding Meaning After Pregnancy Loss*, Kim Hooper and Meredith Resnick, LCSW, with Huong Diep, PsyD

- *The Miscarriage Map Workbook: An Honest Guide to Navigating Pregnancy Loss, Working Through the Pain, and Moving Forward*, Sunita Osborn

- *Not Broken: An Approachable Guide to Miscarriage and Recurrent Pregnancy Loss*, Lora Shahine, MD

- *Your Guide to Miscarriage and Pregnancy Loss: Hope and Healing When You're No Longer Expecting*, Kate White, MD, MPH

Pregnancy and Infant Loss Memoir

- *The Brink of Being: Talking About Miscarriage*, Julia Bueno

- *Ghostbelly*, Elizabeth Heineman

- *What God Is Honored Here?: Writings on Miscarriage and Infant Loss by and for Native Women and Women of Color*, Shannon Gibney and Kao Kalia Yang

Postpartum Care

Please note that postpartum resources typically presume you are postpartum with living children. It may be helpful to keep this in mind as you read. You can take what feels resonant and leave the rest.

- *The First Forty Days: The Essential Art of Nourishing the New Mother*, Heng Ou with Amely Greeven and Marisa Belger
- *The Fourth Trimester: A Postpartum Guide to Healing Your Body, Balancing Your Emotions, and Restoring Your Vitality*, Kimberly Ann Johnson
- *The Fourth Trimester Cards: Daily Support, Inspiration, and Wisdom for New Mothers*, Kimberly Ann Johnson
- *Life After Birth: A Guide to Prepare, Support and Nourish You Through Motherhood*, Jessica Prescott and Vaughne Geary
- *Thriving Postpartum: Embracing the Indigenous Wisdom of La Cuarentena*, Pānquetzani

Motherhood and Female Reproductive Health

- *Essential Labor: Mothering as Social Change*, Angela Garbes
- *Like a Mother: A Feminist Journey Through the Science and Culture of Pregnancy*, Angela Garbes
- *The Pain Gap: How Sexism and Racism in Healthcare Kill Women*, Anushay Hossain
- *Womb: The Inside Story of Where We All Began*, Leah Hazard

Embodied Healing

- *Earth Medicines: Ancestral Wisdom, Healing Recipes, and Wellness Rituals from a Curandera*, Felicia Cocotzin Ruiz
- *Peace of Mind: Becoming Fully Present*, Thich Nhat Hanh
- *Trauma-Informed Yoga Affirmation Card Deck*, Zahabiyah A. Yamasaki with Evelyn Rosario Andry
- *Wild Feminine: Finding Power, Spirit & Joy in the Female Body*, Tami Lynn Kent

Websites

- Association of Women's Health, Obstetric and Neonatal Nurses: awhonn.org/perinatal-bereavement-resources

- CuddleCot: cuddlecot.com

- The Doula Project: nycdoulaproject.org/mab-hotline

- La Leche League: lllusa.org/lactation-after-loss

- The Miscarriage Association: miscarriageassociation.org.uk

- Now I Lay Me Down to Sleep (remembrance photography): nowilaymedowntosleep.org

- Postpartum Support International: postpartum.net

- Pregnancy After Loss Support: pregnancyafterlosssupport.org

- Pregnancy and Infant Loss Support Centre: pilsc.org

- Return to Zero: HOPE: rtzhope.org

- Tommy's: tommys.org

Trainings

- Bereavement Doula: themiscarriagedoula.co

- Holding Space for Pregnancy Loss: birthbreathanddeath.com

- Maternal Mental Health: seleni.org

- Perinatal Mental Health: postpartum.net

Notes

To Tend and To Hold

1. As clarified by Atena Asiaii, MD, MPH, clinically, the term *postpartum* is used after delivery of more than 20 weeks gestation. If your body releases a pregnancy before 20 weeks gestation (with or without intervention), it is typically classified as *postabortion care*. For this book, the term *postpartum* is used to discuss the time after delivery of a pregnancy loss at any point in gestation. Personal interview with Dr. Asiaii on December 3, 2023.

Womb and Womb Loss

1. Atif Ameer Muhammad, Sarah E. Fagan, Jessica N. Sosa-Stanley, Diana C. Peterson, *Anatomy, Abdomen and Pelvis: Uterus* (Florida: StatPearls Publishing, 2022), pubmed.ncbi.nlm.nih.gov/29262069/.

2. "Uterus," Cleveland Clinic, my.clevelandclinic.org/health/body /22467-uterus.

3. Zoey N. Pascual and Michelle D. Langaker, *Physiology, Pregnancy* (Florida: StatPearls Publishing, 2023), ncbi.nlm.nih.gov/books /NBK559304/.

4. "Normal Uterus Size During Pregnancy," American Pregnancy Association, americanpregnancy.org/healthy-pregnancy/pregnancy -health-wellness/uterus-size-during-pregnancy/.

5. "Uterus Involution," Cleveland Clinic, my.clevelandclinic.org/health /articles/22655-uterus-involution.

Introduction: Your Loss Is Our Loss

1. Kathleen Chin, et al., "Suicide and Maternal Mortality," *Current Psychiatry Reports* 24 (April 2022): 239–275, doi.org/10.1007/s11920 -022-01334-3.

2. Lauren A. Kobylski, et al., "Preventing Perinatal Suicide: An Unmet Public Health Need," *The Lancet* 8 (June 2023), thelancet.com /journals/lanpub/article/PIIS2468-2667(23)00092-0/fulltext.

Terminology: A Softer Shared Language

1. "To My Unborn Child," Motherly, December 4, 2020, mother.ly/getting -pregnant/miscarriage-loss/miscarriage-grief-to-my-unborn-child/.

2. As clarified by Atena Asiaii, MD, MPH, since anembryonic pregnancy (also known as a blighted ovum) and biochemical pregnancy (also known as chemical pregnancy) are losses that occur before an intrauterine pregnancy is detected by yolk sac and/or fetal pole, the pregnancy is not established clinically, so trimesters are not applied. Further, clinical debate exists about whether they should be included in the pregnancy count. For this book, they are honored as pregnancies. Personal interview with Dr. Asiaii on December 3, 2023.

3. As clarified by Atena Asiaii, MD, MPH, molar pregnancy is not typically associated with a particular gestational age; it is commonly detected in the first trimester due to abnormal labs or imaging findings. Personal interview with Dr. Asiaii on December 3, 2023.

4. Atena Asiaii, MD, MPH. Personal interview on December 3, 2023.

5. "Stillbirth," National Health Service, nhs.uk/conditions/stillbirth/.

6. "Stillbirth," World Health Organization, who.int/health-topics /stillbirth#tab=tab_1.

Chapter 1: Learning About Your Loss

1. N. S. Macklon, J. P. Geraedts, and B. C. Fauser, "Conception to Ongoing Pregnancy: The 'Black Box' of Early Pregnancy Loss," *Human Reproduction Update* 8, no. 4 (July–August 2002): 333–343, pubmed.ncbi.nlm.nih.gov/12206468/.

2. Nono Simelela, "The Unacceptable Stigma and Shame Women Face After Baby Loss Must End," World Health Organization, who.int/news-room/spotlight/why-we-need-to-talk-about-losing-a-baby/unacceptable-stigma-and-shame.

3. "Newborn Mortality," World Health Organization, January 28, 2022, who.int/news-room/fact-sheets/detail/levels-and-trends-in-child-mortality-report-2021.

4. "Abortion," World Health Organization, November 25, 2021, who.int/news-room/fact-sheets/detail/abortion.

5. Michele Lent Hirsch, "What Is Ambiguous Loss and How to Cope with It?" Everyday Health, October 5, 2022, everydayhealth.com/emotional-health/what-is-ambiguous-loss-and-how-to-cope-with-it/.

6. "Recurrent Pregnancy Loss: Symptoms, Treatment, and Diagnosis," UCLA Health, uclahealth.org/medical-services/obgyn/conditions-treated/recurrent-pregnancy-loss.

7. Atena Asiaii, MD, MPH. Personal interview on December 3, 2023.

Chapter 2: Birthing Your Loss

1. Definition of *birth* from Merriam-Webster, merriam-webster.com/dictionary/birth.

2. Francis Kuehnle, "What to Know About Gender Bias in Healthcare," Medical News Today, October 25, 2021, medicalnewstoday.com/articles/gender-bias-in-healthcare.

3. Crystal Raypole, "Gender Bias in Healthcare Is Very Real—and Sometimes Fatal," Healthline, January 20, 2022, healthline.com/health/gender-bias-healthcare.

4. Layota Hill, Samantha Artiga, and Usha Ranji, "Racial Disparities in Maternal and Infant Health: Current Status and Efforts to Address Them," November 1, 2022, KFF, kff.org/racial-equity-and-health -policy/issue-brief/racial-disparities-in-maternal-and-infant-health -current-status-and-efforts-to-address-them/.

5. Kate White, *Your Guide to Miscarriage & Pregnancy Loss: Hope and Healing When You're No Longer Expecting* (Rochester, MN: Mayo Clinic Press, 2021).

6. "This 'Full Spectrum' Doula Helps with Birth, Miscarriage and Abortion," *Fresh Air*, hosted by Terry Gross, broadcast by National Public Radio, npr.org/2023/04/27/1172200783/this-full-spectrum -doula-helps-with-birth-miscarriage-and-abortion.

Chapter 3: Enduring Your Loss

1. As clarified by Atena Asiaii, MD, MPH, in clinical practice, the term *postpartum* is used only after delivery of more than 20 weeks gestation whereas the term *postabortion care* is used for less than 20 weeks. For this book, the term *postpartum* is used to discuss the time after delivery or the ending of a pregnancy at any gestation. Personal interview on December 3, 2023.

2. "Uterus Involution," Cleveland Clinic, my.clevelandclinic.org/health /diseases/22655-uterus-involution.

3. Sarah Bradley, "What Is Lochia?" Verywell Family, September 21, 2022, verywellfamily.com/what-is-lochia-5079613.

4. Maggie Clark, "Maternal Depression Costs Society Billions Each Year, New Model Finds," Georgetown University McCourt School of Public Policy Center for Children and Families, May 31, 2019, ccf.georgetown.edu/2019/05/31/maternal-depression-costs-society -billions-each-year-new-model-finds/.

5. "How to Deal with Hair Loss After Pregnancy," Cleveland Clinic, June 23, 2022, health.clevelandclinic.org/postpartum-hair-loss.

Chapter 4: Grief in the Postpartum Time

1. "Natural Grief Responses Can Be Seen and Felt Through Many Forms," Our House Grief Support Center, ourhouse-grief.org/grief-pages/grieving-adults/natural-grief-responses/.

2. Jessica Grose, "This Is Your Brain on Motherhood," *The New York Times*, May 5, 2020.

3. Kenneth Doka, "Disenfranchised Grief in Historical and Cultural Perspective," in *Handbook of Bereavement Research and Practice*, ed. M. S. Stroebe, et al., American Psychological Association, APA PsycNet, psycnet.apa.org/record/2008-09330-011.

4. Jenn Morson, "9 Best Heating Pads for Cramps and Menstrual Pain Relief," Healthline, March 30, 2022, healthline.com/health/womens-health/heating-pad-for-cramps.

5. Eleanor Haley, "A Grief Concept You Should Care About: Continuing Bonds," What's Your Grief, February 14, 2018, whatsyourgrief.com/grief-concept-care-continuing-bonds/.

Chapter 5: When Grief and Trauma Intersect

1. Jan Chozen Bays, *Jizo Bodhisattva: Guardian of Children, Travelers, and Other Voyagers* (Boston, MA: Shambhala Publications, 2002).

2. "About Dr. Levine," Ergos Institute of Somatic Education, somaticexperiencing.com/about-peter.

3. "The Toll of Birth Trauma on Your Health," March of Dimes, marchofdimes.org/find-support/topics/postpartum/toll-birth-trauma-your-health.

Chapter 6: Our Loved Ones and Their Grief

1. Nicole Makowka, LMFT. Personal interview on February 13, 2020.

2. "Relaxin," Cleveland Clinic, my.clevelandclinic.org/health/body/24305-relaxin.

Chapter 7: Mourning

1. Dougal Shaw, "The Garden Helping to Heal the Pain of Pregnancy Loss," BBC, June 29, 2019, bbc.com/news/stories-47819487.

Chapter 8: Postpartum Care After Womb Loss

1. Sunita Osborn, *The Miscarriage Map Workbook: An Honest Guide to Navigating Pregnancy Loss, Working Through the Pain, and Moving Forward* (Eau Claire, WI: PESI Publishing, 2021).

2. Diana Cuenca, "Pregnancy Loss: Consequences for Mental Health," *Frontiers in Global Women's Health* 3 (January 23, 2023), doi.org/10.3389/fgwh.2022.1032212.

3. Rhiannon George-Carey, "World Maternal Mental Health Day: Perinatal Mental Health Issues Affect Mothers, Fathers, and Families," Maternal Health Task Force, May 2, 2018, mhtf.org/2018/05/02/world-maternal-mental-health-day-perinatal-mental-health-issues-affect-mothers-fathers-and-families/.

4. Jamila Taylor and Christy M. Gamble, "Suffering in Silence: Mood Disorders Among Pregnant and Postpartum Women of Color," Cap 20, November 17, 2017, americanprogress.org/article/suffering-in-silence/; "Perinatal or Postpartum Mood and Anxiety Disorders," Children's Hospital of Philadelphia, chop.edu/conditions-diseases/perinatal-or-postpartum-mood-and-anxiety-disorders.

5. Christine Mark-Griffin. Personal interview on December 30, 2023.

Chapter 9: How to Support Survivors

1. Definition of *reverence* from Cambridge Dictionary, dictionary.cambridge.org/us/dictionary/english/reverence.

2. Nathan Hodson and Ray Jerram, "Introduction of Miscarriage Bereavement Leave in New Zealand in 2021: A Comparison with International Experiences," *Health Policy* 132 (June 2023), doi.org/10.1016/j.healthpol.2023.104796.

3. Jane Austin. Personal interview on January 3, 2024.

Chapter 10: Returning and Becoming

1. Allan Hall, "The Mother Who Cannot Say Goodbye to Her Dead Child: Tragic Gorilla Cannot Bear to Be Separated from Her Baby a Week After It Died . . . and Still Tries to Wake Her Up," *Daily Mail*, September 17, 2015, dailymail.co.uk/news/article-3238813/The -mother-say-goodbye-dead-child-Tragic-gorilla-bear-separated-baby -week-died-German-zoo-tries-wake-young-daughter.html.

2. Darran Simon, "'Tour of Grief Is Over' for Killer Whale No Longer Carrying Dead Calf," CNN, August 13, 2018, cnn.com/2018/08/12 /us/orca-whale-not-carrying-dead-baby-trnd/index.html.

3. Cynthia Vinney, "Anticipatory Grief Is Actually a Thing— What to Know About It," Verywell Mind, October 23, 2023, verywellmind.com/what-is-anticipatory-grief-5207928.

Contributors

Amanda Griffith Atkins, LMFT, PMHC, is a licensed marriage and family therapist, an Emotions Focused Therapy (EFT) and Eye Movement Desensitization and Reprocessing (EMDR) trained therapist, a certified perinatal mental health therapist, and founder of Amanda Atkins Counseling Group in Chicago. Her clinical specialties are couple's issues, grief and loss, chronic or terminal illness, infertility, postpartum mood disorders, and parenting. She is especially passionate about addressing complex demands placed on parents of disabled children and is herself a mom of a disabled child.

amandagriffithatkins.com | @amanda.griffith.atkins

Marisa Belger is dedicated to supporting women at every stage of the motherhood journey. She is a motherhood coach, women's circle facilitator, and coauthor of bestselling books for mothers, including *The First Forty Days: The Essential Art of Nourishing the New Mother*, the beloved guide to women-centric care in the early weeks of motherhood. She helps women tune into the wisdom of their inner knowing to make the best choices for their peace and fulfillment.

marisabelger.com | @marisabelger

Katrina dela Cruz, MSW, LCSW, CYI, is a psychotherapist, spiritual coach, counselor, plant spiritist, herbalist, energy and sound healer, and Womb Keeper in the Munay-Ki tradition. After over a decade as a hospital clinician, including on OB/GYN and L&D units, Katrina started her private practice, Fire Moon Medicines, where she integrates Western psychological theory with alternative, Indigenous, and ancestral healing traditions. She is especially drawn to the beginning and end of life and the incredible privilege of holding space during these times. She is a womb loss survivor—mother to two spirit babies, Zeo Thomas Farr and Solis Vida Farr.

firemoonmedicines.com | @firemoonmedicines

Jenna Furnari, MA, CAP, holds a master of arts in Ayurveda, is a board-certified Ayurvedic practitioner, Ayurvedic postpartum specialist and trainer, DONA-trained postpartum doula, and founder of Ayurvedic Mamas. Since deep impressions that can last a lifetime are set in the first six weeks following birth, Jenna's intention is to reach as many women as possible with complete care and support through the first 42 days of motherhood. She created the Ayurvedic Postpartum Doula Online Training, bringing this education to hundreds of women worldwide. She lives in Los Angeles, California, with her husband and three children.

jennafurnari.com | @ayurvedic_mamas

Michelle Goebel-Angel, LAc, MSOM, Dipl Ac (NCCAOM), MBA, is a licensed Traditional Chinese Medicine and acupuncture provider at the Raby Institute for Integrative Medicine at Northwestern in Chicago. Michelle is known for her enthusiasm and warmth, and is committed to providing treatments that support the body's natural ability to rebalance and heal itself. She draws from her decades-plus study of essential oils, integrating them into and elevating her treatments. As a mother to three living children and a womb loss survivor, she understands and has a deep reverence for the processes of conception, pregnancy, labor, birth, and postpartum healing; she is ardent in her support for all who endure them.

michelleangelacupuncture.com | rabyintegrativemedicine.com

Kiley Krekorian Hanish, OTD, PMH-C, is the founding director of Return to Zero: HOPE, a national nonprofit organization dedicated to offering support and resources to bereaved families after pregnancy and infant loss. She is also co-creator of the Emmy-nominated film *Return to Zero*, which is based on her experience of womb loss with her son, Norbert, who was still-born at 35 weeks. As a neurodivergent occupational therapist specializing in mental health during the perinatal period, she is passionate about working with bereaved families to help them find purpose, meaning, and healing after pregnancy and infant loss.

rtzhope.org | @rtzhope

Sparrow Harrington, CEIM, CMT, is a certified massage therapist and authorized instructor of prenatal and perinatal massage therapy, certified Mercier therapist, certified educator of infant massage, birth and full-spectrum doula, and founder and owner of Sparrow's Nest, a pregnancy care center in Los Angeles. Sparrow has witnessed the profound impact that skilled, nurturing touch plays in healing after the deepest loss and hopes to see postpartum bereavement massage become a well-known and widely available offering.

sparrowmassage.com | @sparrows_nest_massage

Molly Boeder Harris, MA, E-RYT, SEP, is a Somatic Experiencing® Practitioner, trauma-informed yoga teacher, and the founder of The Breathe Network—a national nonprofit that connects survivors of sexual trauma with trauma-informed, holistic healing practitioners and also offers trauma-informed care training in health-care and healing spaces. Molly is a mother to her beautiful child and is a womb loss survivor.

mollyboederharris.com | @thebreathenetwork

Lucy Kupferstein, CHC, is a certified integrative nutrition coach and an Associate Acutonics practitioner. After the death of her son, Sig, in utero at fifteen weeks gestation due to a preterm premature membrane rupture, she turned to food to heal her womb from the inside out. This inspired her to shift her work to support women navigating the profound journey of fertility. Lucy specializes in nutrition coaching for pre-conception and is passionate about empowering women with the knowledge of how food can nurture a healthy womb environment.

thedenofmuses.com | @denofmuseswellness

Nicole Longmire, MPH, IBCLC, PMH-C, is an International Board Certified Lactation Consultant, certified Birth Story Listener, childbirth educator, postpartum doula, and Holding Space Facilitator. She is the founder of Mother Nurture Consulting, where she helps families prepare for and navigate the journey to parenthood, including helping mothers successfully breastfeed their earth-side babies. She also specializes in working with women who have experienced pregnancy and infant loss, traumatic birth, and breastfeeding grief, supporting them with lactation after loss. She is a mom to her living son, two bonus sons, and her forever baby Owen, who was born in 2021, lived for 36 days, and died from complications due to CCHD.

mothernurturelactationservices.com | @motheringnurtured

Princess Estocia McKinney is an author, birth-postpartum doula, mother of two living children, and a womb loss survivor. She is passionate about helping those who are postpartum feel held in the loving embrace that belly wrapping can provide and does so through her company, Bellibind, which offers in-person belly-binding services, wrap kits with virtual self-binding guidance, training for birth workers who want to learn the ancient art of Bengkung belly binding, and gifted sessions to survivors of womb loss.

bellibind.com | @bellibind

Yiska Obadia, LAc, is a licensed acupuncturist, bodyworker, certified Havening practitioner, and DONA-trained birth doula. With birth and touch as two of her greatest passions, she created *Comforting Touch for Birth*, a comprehensive curriculum for birth and postpartum doulas and expectant parents to learn how to share deeply supportive touch with their clients and pregnant partners. She is also the creator of the *Wisdom of Birth* oracle deck, offering guidance and inspiration for pregnant people and their families. After years of navigating fertility challenges, Yiska is now a loving foster mother.

yiskaobadia.com | @comfortingtouchdoula

Heng Ou is an author, mother of three, and founder of the Los Angeles-based global motherhood support platform MotherBees. After her first birth, she practiced zuo yuezi, a traditional Chinese approach to postpartum care passed down to her by cherished family members. Deeply moved by the rejuvenating power of this practice, Heng felt compelled to make it accessible to a broader audience and started a postpartum food delivery service that has since grown into an international hive of connection, experiences, and education for mothers. She is the author of the seminal book *The First Forty Days: The Essential Art of Nourishing the New Mother,* which has helped to center postpartum care in the United States and beyond since its release in 2016. She is also the author of *Nine Golden Months: The Essential Art of Nurturing the Mother-to-Be* and *Awakening Fertility: The Essential Art of Preparing for Pregnancy.*

motherbees.com | @motherbees.

Nora Vitaliani is a San Francisco-based chef and caterer specializing in honoring the wisdom and healing power of seasonal foods. Nora is highly regarded for the care she devotes to choosing high-quality ingredients and her intuitive gift for cooking that inspires a deep-felt sense of being nourished and cared for. She has been supporting bereaved mothers since 2021, when she began catering Return to Zero: HOPE's holistic retreats for those who have experienced pregnancy and infant loss.

justeatitsf.com | @just_eat_it_sf

Betsy Winter is a mind-body coach, perinatal grief and trauma somatic specialist, Nia Black Belt instructor, director of community support for Return to Zero: HOPE, and a womb loss survivor. She has been providing trauma-informed, holistic, and inclusive support and resources for bereaved parents since 2015, when her daughter, Eliza, died in utero at 41 weeks due to hypoplastic left heart syndrome and trisomy 18. She is known for her heart-centered approach to healing and transforming pain from trauma, grief, loss, and early childhood wounding.

betsywinter.com | rtzhope.org

Zahabiyah (Zabie) Yamasaki, MEd, RYT, is a sought-after trauma-informed yoga teacher, educator, national trainer, keynote speaker, and the founder of

Transcending Sexual Trauma Through Yoga, an organization with the mission of empowering survivors to heal through the practice of yoga. Zabie is also the author of *Trauma-Informed Yoga for Survivors of Sexual Assault*, *Trauma-Informed Yoga Affirmation Deck*, *Trauma-Informed Yoga Flip Chart*, *Your Joy Is Beautiful*, and *H Is for Healing Card Deck*. She is a mother to a living child and a womb loss survivor.

zabieyamasaki.com | @transcending_trauma_with_yoga

About the Artist

J o Situ Allen, also known as DIRTY ERASER, is a California artist known for her dreamy and high-frequency multimedia works and paintings that transport the viewer into the energetics of the natural world. Jo's offerings are guided by her intuitive sense of social and ecological harmony, informed by her bachelor's and master's degrees in geography and sustainability. Jo is sought out for her work as a visual dreamer, creative director, and storyteller, merging the worlds of science, spirit, and art. She is the author of two books on California's native species.

dirtyeraser.com | @dirty_eraser

About the Author

Eileen Santos Rosete, MSMFT, PCD(DONA), CYT 200, holds a master of science in marriage and family therapy from Northwestern University and is certified as a DONA International postpartum doula, trauma-informed yoga teacher, and grief educator. Her brand, Our Sacred Women®, is known for its elevated offerings that help women feel seen, held, and honored. She is especially passionate about supporting those who are postpartum—both after live births and after loss. Eileen is known for her warmth and intuitive ability to hold space with compassion. She has been leading grief support groups at Our House Grief Support Center in Los Angeles since 2019, where she completed advanced professional training. Her work is inspired by simple yet profound moments of feeling witnessed and at ease in her body, as well as her longing to help others feel the same. She lives with her husband and three living children in California.

eileensantosrosete.com | @oursacredwomen

About Sounds True

Sounds True was founded in 1985 by Tami Simon with a clear mission: to disseminate spiritual wisdom. Since starting out as a project with one woman and her tape recorder, we have grown into a multimedia publishing company with a catalog of more than 3,000 titles by some of the leading teachers and visionaries of our time, and an ever-expanding family of beloved customers from across the world.

In more than three decades of evolution, Sounds True has maintained our focus on our overriding purpose and mission: to wake up the world. We offer books, audio programs, online learning experiences, and in-person events to support your personal growth and awakening, and to unlock our greatest human capacities to love and serve.

At SoundsTrue.com you'll find a wealth of resources to enrich your journey, including our weekly *Insights at the Edge* podcast, free downloads, and information about our nonprofit Sounds True Foundation, where we strive to remove financial barriers to the materials we publish through scholarships and donations worldwide.

To learn more, please visit SoundsTrue.com/freegifts or call us toll-free at 800.333.9185.

Together, we can wake up the world.

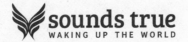